History as Evidence

Nursing Interventions Through Time

Patricia D'Antonio, PhD, RN, FAAN, is currently an Associate Professor of Nursing, the Associate Director of the Barbara Bates Center for the Study of the History of Nursing University of Pennsylvania, and a Fellow of the American Academy of Nursing. She is also the editor of the *Nursing History Review*, the official journal of the American Association for the History of Nursing. Her work on early nineteenth-century psychiatric care has been published in her book, *Founding Friends: Families, Staff, and Patients at the Friends Asylum in Early Nineteenth Century Philadelphia.* Her most recent research on the history of American nursing has been published as *American Nursing: A History of Knowledge, Authority and the Meaning of Work.* Her awards include a National Humanities Foundation Fellowship, the Penn Humanities Forum Mellon Faculty Research Fellowship, the National Library of Medicine Grant for Scholarly Works, Best of the *Journal of Nursing Scholarship*—Profession and Society, the Barbara Brodie Nursing History Fellowship from the University of Virginia, and the Lavinia Dock Award from the American Association for the History of Nursing. Her books *Enduring Issues in American Nursing* (co-edited), *Founding Friends,* and *Nurses Work: Issues Across Time and Place* (co-edited) have received the *American Journal of Nursing*'s Book of the Year award. She serves on the advisory boards of the UK Centre for the History of Nursing and Midwifery and the International Network for Nursing History and Thinking in Madrid.

Sandra B. Lewenson, EdD, RN, FAAN, integrates nursing's rich history into her teaching as Professor of Nursing at the Lienhard School of Nursing, Pace University in New York. Dr. Lewenson has received several awards throughout her career, including the Outstanding Scholarship and Research Award from Teachers College, Columbia University, induction into the Hall of Fame of the Alumni Association of Hunter College, Pace University Keenan Award for Teaching Excellence, and the American Association for the History of Nursing Lavinia Dock Award for Historical Scholarship and Research in Nursing for her seminal work, *Taking Charge: Nursing, Suffrage, and Feminism in America, 1873–1920.* She also received two *American Journal of Nursing* Book of the Year awards for *Capturing Nursing History: A Guide to Historical Methods in Research* and *Decision-Making in Nursing: Thoughtful Approaches for Practice.* Dr. Lewenson is a member of the American Academy of Nursing and Sigma Theta Tau International Honor Society. She recently co-edited *Public Health Nursing: Practicing Population-Based Care.*

History as Evidence

Nursing Interventions Through Time

Patricia D'Antonio, PhD, RN, FAAN

Sandra B. Lewenson, EdD, RN, FAAN

SPRINGER PUBLISHING COMPANY
NEW YORK

Springer Publishing Company, LLC
11 West 42nd Street
New York, NY 10036
www.springerpub.com

Acquisitions Editor: Allan Graubard
Cover Design: David Levy
Composition: S4Carlisle Publishing Services

ISBN: 978-0-8261-0577-6

10 11 12/ 5 4 3 2 1

The author and the publisher of this Work have made every effort to use sources believed to be reliable to provide information that is accurate and compatible with the standards generally accepted at the time of publication. Because medical science is continually advancing, our knowledge base continues to expand. Therefore, as new information becomes available, changes in procedures become necessary. We recommend that the reader always consult current research and specific institutional policies before performing any clinical procedure. The author and publisher shall not be liable for any special, consequential, or exemplary damages resulting, in whole or in part, from the readers' use of, or reliance on, the information contained in this book. The publisher has no responsibility for the persistence or accuracy of URLs for external or third-party Internet Web sites referred to in this publication and does not guarantee that any content on such Web sites is, or will remain, accurate or appropriate.

Library of Congress Cataloging-in-Publication Data

History as evidence: nursing interventions through time / [edited by]
Patricia D'Antonio, Sandra B. Lewenson.
p. ; cm.
Includes bibliographical references and index.
ISBN 978-0-8261-0577-6
1. Nursing—History. 2. Evidence-based nursing. I. D'Antonio, Patricia,
1955– II. Lewenson, Sandra.
[DNLM: 1. Evidence-Based Nursing—history. 2. History of Nursing. WY 11.1]
RT31.H567 2010
610.73—dc22

2010028860

Printed in the United States of America by Hamilton Printing Company

We dedicate this book to Karen Buhler-Wilkerson, who taught so many of us to do historical research and to appreciate and learn from the nurses who came before us.

Contents

Contributors

Rima D. Apple, PhD Professor Emerita, University of Wisconsin-Madison, Madison, Wisconsin

J. Margo Brooks Carthon, PhD, RN Post Doctoral Fellow, Barbara Bates Center for the Study of the History of Nursing, Center for Health Outcomes and Policy Research, University of Pennsylvania School of Nursing, Philadelphia, Pennsylvania

Joy Buck, PhD, APRN Associate Professor, West Virginia University School of Nursing and Department of Family Medicine, Eastern Division, Morgantown, West Virginia

Kathleen G. Burke, PhD, RN Practice Assistant Professor, and Director, Nursing and Healthcare Administration and Healthcare Leadership Programs, University of Pennsylvania School of Nursing, Philadelphia, Pennsylvania

Cynthia Anne Connolly, PhD, RN, PNP Associate Professor, University of Pennsylvania School of Nursing, Philadelphia, Pennsylvania

Julie A. Fairman, PhD, FAAN, RN Professor and Director, Barbara Bates Center for the Study of the History of Nursing, University of Pennsylvania School of Nursing, Philadelphia, Pennsylvania

Karen Flynn, PhD Assistant Professor, Gender & Women's Studies Program, University of Illinois, Urbana-Champaign, Champaign, Illinois

Arlene Keeling, PhD, FAAN, RN The Centennial Distinguished Professor of Nursing Directory, The Center for Nursing Historical Inquiry, The University of Virginia School of Nursing, Charlottesville, Virginia

Brigid Lusk, PhD, RN Chair and Professor, Northern Illinois University School of Nursing and Health Studies, DeKalb, Illinois

Sylvia Rinker, PhD, RN Professor Emerita, Lynchburg College, Lynchburg, Virginia

Linda Sabin, RNC, PHD Professor, University of Louisiana at Monroe School of Nursing, Monroe, Louisiana

Barbra Mann Wall, PhD, RN Associate Professor and Associate Director, Barbara Bates Center for the Study of the History of Nursing, University of Pennsylvania School of Nursing, Philadelphia, Pennsylvania

Lisa M. Zerull, PhD, RN, FCN Academic Liaison and Program Manager, Winchester Medical Center/Valley Health, Winchester, Virginia

Helen Zuelzer, RN, MS, NP, CWOCN Doctoral Student, University of Virginia School of Nursing, Charlottesville, Virginia

Foreword

The power of a story to entice and capture an individual's interest and imagination has been amply demonstrated over the centuries by the popularity of story tellers, novels, plays, and movies in society. From antiquity to the present, people have sought opportunities to vicariously enter into the lives of others to learn what they think and do, and what happens to the people in the story as a result of life's events. The timeless issues that surround human illness are often found in stories because authors have always recognized the inherent drama that occurs when an individual is born, becomes ill, and dies. From such stories, nurses have opportunities to learn more about the range of human experiences and information they might incorporate in their care of patients.

For those interested in learning more about the antecedents of today's health care and what nurses contributed to the development of modern health care, *History as Evidence: Nursing Interventions Through Time* is a veritable gold mine of thoughtful and stimulating historical studies. Many of the studies, which trace how nurses used their talents to develop ways to render effective nursing care to patients, read as stories because they tell how nurses kept abreast of advances in medicine and used this information to care for their patients, alleviate their suffering, and help them remain healthy. The studies also reveal how professional nurses expanded their view of nursing from the patient's bedside to become health care leaders and innovators who developed effective medical therapies, and aided health policy makers in developing more equitable health policies.

The diversity of the subjects discussed reveals that medical and nursing practices were always defined by what was scientifically known and understood about the etiology and pathophysiology of diseases and what had been found to be effective in treating medical problems. Each generation of scientists and health professionals added to this body of medical knowledge as they strove to devise new medical interventions in hopes that they could improve the lives of patients. Linda Sabin's study on the medical care of yellow fever patients in the nineteenth century vividly depicts what physicians understood about the origin and manifestation of the disease, and what were the methods they used to treat patients and stop the spread of the fever. Readers may be surprised to learn how quickly fever patients could die, the strange treatments used by physicians to try to save those stricken, and, finally, that it was good nursing care that the made the difference in whether fever patients lived or died. After reading this chapter, readers will recognize the tremendous advances in medical science that were made in the twentieth century that allow today's health professionals the scientific knowledge and technology needed to successfully treat many of today's medical problems.

The book's historical studies include the care of patients with tuberculosis, cancer, vexing bedsores, and influenza in the epidemic of 1915. They also include stories about the development of hospice nursing and public health services in rural America. As a whole, these stories provide readers with sharp clinical details of how patients suffered from the ravages of diseases, and what were the nursing interventions used by nurses to help patients regain their health. Brigid Lusk's chapter on the nursing of patients with cancer during the 1950s is an excellent example of the richness of these stories. Lusk captures both the radical and often disfiguring surgeries and medical therapy employed to rid patients of their malignancies, and the struggles of nurses to emotionally and physically support these patients through their hospitalization and when at home with their families. Her insights into what enabled nurses to become creative in developing effective ways to treat the side effects of the new cancer interventions and why nurses demanded for a voice in the debate about whether patients should be informed that they had cancer are especially poignant and enlightening. She concludes that, no matter how complex the patient's medical therapy might become, nurses must not be diverted from being strong advocates for their patients.

The introduction of complex medical technology in the care of patients is addressed in Kathleen Burke's study as she explores how technology expanded the ability of physicians to medically manage patients' problems and how it also broadened the role and practice of acute care nurses. The introduction of the Swan-Ganz ctheter in a surgical intensive care unit in the 1970s serves as wonderful example of how essential nurses were in evaluating and adapting this technology to meet the needs of patients. Given little information about how the catheter worked, nurses were faced with the challenge of caring for patients with the devise inserted in their heart. Using historical records and oral interviews of nurses who worked in the unit at the time, Burke provides a window into this SICU, and documents how adaptable and independent nurses were in modifying the medical technology to assure that it helped their patients. Burke demonstrates that the nurses' professional experience and medical knowledge enabled them to incorporate this new technology into their practice, and in doing so, they enlarged their clinical responsibilities and became more autonomous in making clinical decisions about patients. As they became more knowledgeable and medically proficient, the relationship between physicians and nurses also changed. The staff recognized that patients received better care when they functioned as a medical team, and that included jointly developing the unit's medical protocols for the care of their patients.

Barbra Mann Wall's study on the contributions of Catholic sister-nurses to the care of patients and the development of hospitals adds an important perspective in our understanding of the diversity of the nurses that created and shaped the nursing profession. Catholic sister-nurses shared the commitment of secular nurses to provide patients care that was based on the most current scientific knowledge available. Yet sister-nurses also believed that there was a powerful spiritual dimension of care beyond that found in modern scientific medicine. And they believed that this spiritual dimension was especially beneficial to patients when they were seriously ill and in danger of death. Catholic hospitals were designed to reflect the presence of God throughout the hospital, including patients' rooms and the chapel. A religious atmosphere was sustained in the hospital by daily prayer services, devotions, and through the use of sacraments. It was also incorporated into the daily lives of the staff and patients. Treading a delicate path of providing spiritual aid to those who believe in the spiritual life of man and, at the same time, not wishing to proselytize those who did not, the sister-nurses provided all patients modern medical care delivered by professional physicians and nurses. Over time, modern medicine has come to recognize the spiritual aspects of the human experience and many health care professionals now incorporate dimensions of spirituality into their practice. In addition, as Lisa Zerull points out in her story, a new nursing role has been created: parish nursing. Parish nurses serve a religious community by offering church members opportunities to obtain health advice and counseling that integrates medical knowledge with spirituality.

One of the more intriguing stories to me is Helen Zuelzer's study of how nurses and physicians attempted to prevent and care for patients' bedsores. In her careful review of nursing literature from the late 1800s to the 1940s, Zuelzer documents not only the multiple treatments used by experts to prevent and treat bedsores, but also that the experts always believed that some patients' bedsores were neither preventable nor treatable. The advent of antimicrobial treatments began in the late 1940s, and the additional knowledge learned about the pathophysiology and treatment of pressure ulcers has led to much more success in preventing and healing this "obstinate sore." But the intriguing question I am left with is: Will we find, as did other nurses before us, that there are some patients whose pressure ulcers are not amenable to therapy, especially in the population of older frail patients who lack the ability to regenerate new tissue? This is an important nursing question especially in light of Medicare's recent decision that places the cost of treating patients who develop one while hospitalized on the institution itself. Further study of hospitals' ability to prevent and treat patients with pressure sores should produce data that either sustains the government's assumption that pressure ulcers are the result of inadequate nursing care or prove that there are some inherent differences in individuals that lead to the appearance of pressure sores.

Nurses should read *History as Evidence: Nursing Interventions Through Time* for three reasons: the book is compelling and interesting to read; it attests to the legacy of nurses in being able to provide competent and compassionate care to the sick; and it charts their essential role in the health care system. It also offers evidence of the ability of nursing history to stimulate nurses to think about their practice and role in the health system in a different light. It offers valuable insights into the forces that shaped yesterday's and today's nurses and the quality of care that they provide the public. Nursing's history captures not only what nursing care was like in the past but also why it was done, and more importantly, whether this care added to nursing's body of knowledge. In the end, studying nursing's history offers faculty and students an attractive and effective method to stimulate learning beyond the facts to be studied. In analyzing and discussing the reasons for nursing measures used in the past, we can all become more competent in clinical practice, better able to navigate the frequent changes that occur in the health system, and committed to a tradition of providing competent and compassionate care to patients.

Barbara Brodie, PhD, RN, FAAN
Professor Emerita
Associate Director, Center for Nursing Historical Inquiry
University of Virginia School of Nursing
Charlottesville, Virginia
bb9w@virginia.edu

Preface

An increasing emphasis on evidence-based practice promises to transform what clinicians do for their patients, how clinicians think about and solve problems present in practice, and, in the end, what clinicians consider the dimensions of "good" patient care. Once we believed that standards of evidence might be found only in rigorously controlled double-blind clinical trials. These remain the "gold standard" of evidence, but we now know that many other sources of evidence exist. They may lie in an increasing body of literature pointing to the efficacy of a certain intervention. They may also survive in the clinical wisdom of an experienced practitioner responding to the reality of a clinical crisis. And they may be present within the relationships in particular practices where some clinicians have more power than others to decide what actually constitutes evidence.

In *History as Evidence: Nursing Interventions Through Time* we show how historical practices, policies, and procedures also serve as evidence for current practice. In some ways, we return to an earlier tradition of practice where searches for what might work in the present would be found in the wisdom of the writings of ancient masters. But in *History as Evidence: Nursing Interventions Through Time* we move beyond drawing simplistic associations and encourage readers to think critically about practices in time and place. In each chapter in this edited collection, we invite authors who are specialists in the histories of different clinical nursing specialties to use their data to answer a specific set of questions that will guide readers through this process. How did particular nursing interventions come about? Why did particular nursing interventions come about? What parts of these interventions remain with us? What parts have been shed? What has been gained? What has been lost? And, finally, how might these particular stories inform the ways in which we evaluate contemporary standards?

History as Evidence: Nursing Interventions Through Time provides one of the first responses to the American Association of Colleges of Nursing's (AACN) new *Essentials of Baccalaureate Nursing Education.* The *Essentials* are clear in the AACN's intent that these programs more successfully integrate the liberal arts into nursing education. This has often proved challenging. Our edited book uses history, one of the most prominent of the liberal arts, and explicitly links the insights gained in this field to current clinical practice. We anticipate that it will bring together readers' disparate backgrounds and unite them in the process of discovering how one liberal art can help them in the process of evaluating, critiquing, and, perhaps, transforming practice. To paraphrase what one of the co-editors wrote in another venue, we present these histories of practice as an exemplar of how the liberal arts can help students more fully understand and respond to the complexities, the ambiguities, and the keenly felt sense of responsibility that characterize nursing interventions in the past as well as in the present.[1]

The history of nursing unfolds in a unique way as historians study the context of nursing interventions over time. Nurses cared for the sick, sought ways to assist the dying, participated in new ways to treat childbirth, instituted innovative technologies in care, collaborated in the treatment of epidemics, negotiated space in which to practice, and advocated policies that would provide care for populations in need. Their stories add a new dimension to the historical record. The interventions of nurses working in various specialties and settings throughout the nineteenth and twentieth centuries contributed to the changing landscape of health care in the United States. Often unrecognized for their contributions, these stories highlight nursing interventions over time and offer insight into not only what nurses did in the past, but what they can do today.

History as Evidence: Nursing Interventions Through Time introduces the reader to why an historical understanding of nursing interventions has an important place in current practice. Taken as a whole, the chapters in this book highlight how some practice issues, such as pressure ulcers or safety, have been longstanding issues in nursing practice; and they emphasize how some practice populations, such as children or vulnerable men and women, have always been within nursing's domain. These chapters also attend to the importance of context to nursing interventions. The processes of deciding what constitutes evidence for practice has always and still exists within influential social, political, racial, and gender contexts that are sometimes as important as data. They highlight the often-ignored question: What did nurses actually do to care for their patients in the past? And finally, these chapters explore how interventions should not be understood as antiquated practices, but as sometimes effective responses that can be mined for their ability to reconstruct current practices. *Nursing History* provides an important tool that brings together a body of knowledge about past practice while presenting a new perspective on the interpretation of nurses'

---

[1]Patricia D'Antonio, Ellen D. Baer, Sylvia D. Rinker, and Joan E. Lynaugh, eds. *Nurses' Work: Issues Across Time and Place* (New York: Springer), 2001.

work. Without an understanding of the work nurses have done, the worth of nursing's important and successful interventions are lost.

INTRODUCTION TO THE CHAPTERS

History as Evidence: Nursing Interventions Through Time uses both time and context to organize the chapters into four sections. The first section, *Nursing Interventions: Providing Care*, explores the procedures nurses used when treating those affected by various diseases and conditions. It provides examples of how nurses cared for patients sick with yellow fever, how they treated children who were infected with tuberculosis (TB), how they responded to the overwhelming influenza pandemic, and how they treated patients who developed bedsores (and the nursing interventions used to prevent them from occurring). Nursing interventions changed over time in response to such factors as availability of caregivers, seemingly uncontrollable spread of disease, and increasing scientific knowledge.

The second section, *Nursing Interventions: Offering Service*, presents histories that look at the nursing work provided to specific populations that might not have received care. The chapters in this section look at the kind of nursing care offered by nursing sisters, community activists, and denomination-based parish nurses. These nurses infused their care with an additional purpose that served the needs of particularly vulnerable populations. Their nursing interventions integrated social consciousness, spirituality, and missionary zeal to provide care during the early half of the twentieth century.

The third section, *Nursing Interventions: Influencing Change*, examines nurses' ability to accept, influence, and support the use of innovations in practice during the mid-twentieth century. Here we see how nurses have adapted to change and influenced the diffusion of change as new medical practices and technologies emerged throughout the twentieth century. Chapters in this section explore how accepting scientific principles significantly altered the meanings attributed to the birthing process and the care offered to cancer patients. They also show the contextual influences that came into play in the adoption of life-saving technology in the intensive care units and how these influences also occurred in a racialized and gendered environment. Most important, these chapters show how nurses were active agents in the process of change: They were neither victims of the technological imperatives nor passive spectators only following medical orders.

And finally, the fourth section, *Nursing Interventions: Negotiating Space,* discuss two issues: (1) the tension nurses have experienced in their relationships with physicians and the public and (2) the ways in which nursing interventions take on a broad range of activities that speak to and move beyond that tension. In order to promote health throughout the life span and support patients in need of care, nurses negotiated spaces in which they practiced. They demonstrated the efficacy of public health nurses in a community. They negotiated professional practice agreements as a nurse practitioner. And they advocated for appropriate end-of-life care. This was not always easy, and historical evidence into the challenges that nurses faced as they carved out new roles and space in which to practice offers an important perspective to consider today.

Although we have placed chapters within various sections, we acknowledge that the overarching threads of continuity, context, and actual practice can come together and pull apart in many other kinds of ways as well. In addition, issues related to power, negotiation, space, politics, gender, race, and economics often emerge in each chapter regardless of context or, for that matter, chronology. Nursing history cannot be separated from the larger context in which nurses have practiced over time. But the pieces of that history that may have the most relevance for a particular reader may be different from that presented in our particular organizational framework. We encourage readers to not only read the chapters as a whole, but to also move back and forth between chapters that seem to have the most salience for them and their practice. To that end, we present a summary of the main foci of each chapter in *Nursing History: Interventions through Time.*

NURSING INTERVENTIONS: PROVIDING CARE

In Chapter 1, *Sweating, Purging, and a Passion for Care: The Yellow Fever Nurse in the Deep South in the Early Nineteenth Century*, Linda Sabin examines the actual interventions nurses provided during the yellow fever outbreaks in the Deep South during the first half of the nineteenth century. Long before the opening of formal nurse training schools in the United States, caregivers learned their skill by experience alone. Sabin also explores the contextual factors that these early nurses faced as they provided care. The warm, moist environment of the Deep South, the social and political institution of slavery, the harsh medical treatments available at the time, and the lack of hygiene and sanitation affected nursing interventions. Caregivers implemented the medical treatments of the day as they administered hot mustard baths, laxatives, and cool baths to reduce fever. Sabin's work shows the critical impact these men and women had on their family and their community's survival. These nineteenth-century caregivers who faced the many challenges presented by fever nursing may serve, Sabin suggests, as role models for caregivers facing epidemics today.

Cynthia Anne Connolly moves us into the early twentieth century in the next chapter, *Determining Children's "Best Interests" in the Midst of an Epidemic: A Cautionary Tale From History.* Connolly writes about nurses and the preventorium, an early twentieth-century institution designed to prevent the emergence of active TB in poor children who had tested positive to the newly developed tuberculin test. With the discovery of the tuberculin test came a movement to save these newly diagnosed "pretubercular" children before any symptoms of the disease appeared. This movement established preventoria throughout the country that took poor "pretubucular" children from their own homes and placed them in institutions run by nurses. Connolly uses the Farmingdale Tuberculosis Preventorium for Children, opened in 1909, to explore the issues surrounding this intervention for children and the meaning it has for us today. Issues such as interdisciplinary collaboration, difficulty in translating new research into practice, intersecting boundaries of the rights of the public, children, and family, ethnic or class-based bias are important to consider in light of the current issues that surround children and health care today, and, in particular, the epidemic of obesity that focuses on the bodies of poorer children across the United States.

In *Treating Influenza 1918 and 2010: Recycled Interventions,* Arlene W. Keeling looks at the kinds of enduring interventions nurses used to treat influenza during the pandemic of 1918 through a historical account of the ravages wrought by that pandemic. The staggering loss of life, particularly of young adults worldwide at a time the world was dealing with the crisis of World War I, necessitated extraordinary measures from public health nurses to combat the pandemic. Keeling shows how nursing care served as the primary treatment for influenza in 1918. Interventions such as sponging patients reduced fevers; opening windows and offering soups and nourishment offered some relief to the victims. Nurses responded to the pandemic in urban and rural communities offering public health education among the interventions they offered. Keeling provides historical evidence that links the response to H1N1 in 2010 with the earlier pandemic in 1918 and suggests the enduring necessity of excellent nursing care.

Concern about pressure ulcers remains a topic of discussion that has lasted well over a century. Helen Zuelzer studies the historical evidence surrounding the nursing care of what were then called bedsores in, *"An Obstinate and Sometimes Gangrenous Sore": Prevention and Nursing Care of Bedsores, 1900 to the 1940s.* This chapter relates the relevance of bedsores and the nursing interventions used to prevent and treat them with the new federal legislation that promises to hold acute care settings accountable if patients develop them.

Zuelzer explores the treatment and prevention of bedsores using what was written in the nursing literature between 1900 and 1940. Prevention of sores remained essentially the nurses' responsibility: that meant keeping the bed sheets smooth, the skin dry, and patients frequently turned and positioned. The question of whether all bedsores could be prevented engendered much controversy and remained unanswered. Change in treatments over time reflected the knowledge nurses gained from experience, a process that continues today.

NURSING INTERVENTIONS: OFFERING SERVICE

Barbara Mann Wall's chapter, *Body, Soul, and Service: Catholic Sister-Nurses in Late Nineteenth and Early Twentieth Century Hospitals*, examines the work of three religious orders as they integrated spirituality into their nursing care. Wall shows how sister-nurses blended religious activities with scientific nursing practices—practices that resulted in greater access to care and better care for patients. Chapels built inside the hospitals served as a space where sister-nurses could combine nursing with religious interventions. Nuns followed medical orders, but they did so as they followed their religious mission to help dying patients who were Catholic, or potential Catholics, achieve what Wall describes as "penance, resignation, and prayer." The work of these sister-nuns during the late-nineteenth and early-twentieth centuries provides case studies that nurses might use today when integrating the mind, body, and spirit into the care they provide.

Set in the city of Philadelphia, J. Margo Brooks Carthon's chapter, *Bridging the Gaps: Collaborative Health Work in the City of Brotherly Love, 1900–1920*, examines the efforts of the Black community to provide much-needed health care services to underserved populations. Brooks Carthon uses historical evidence about how this community—socially, politically, and economically marginalized—developed a system to support members in need. The lack of social services available to the large number of Black families who immigrated from the South to Philadelphia in search of jobs and a better life led to overcrowded living conditions. Black community leaders feared the spread of infectious diseases, especially TB. Without much hope of receiving the necessary public health services, the Whittier Centre, a philanthropic group organized in 1912 by Black and White community activists, considered ways in which to address the disease. One solution was to hire a Black public health nurse, Elizabeth Tyler, to identify cases of TB in the Black community. Brooks Carthon's study reveals that the combined work of these civic activists and public health nurses led to the eventual expansion of health promotion and disease prevention services, pointing to the continued need of strong community support for necessary health prevention work.

In the next chapter, *Filling the Gaps in Community Care: Parish Nurses Working Out of Congregations*, Lisa M. Zerull considers faith-based nursing as a possible solution to our own much-needed community health services. Zerull studies the history of deaconess nurses associated with the Baltimore Lutheran Deaconess Motherhouse in Baltimore, Maryland, during the early part of the twentieth century. Deaconess nurses, a new role for women in the church at that time, included spiritual care and social service among the nursing interventions they brought to the urban poor as they were trained to care for the soul as well as the body. Zerull points to the history of faith-based nursing services as a way for current practitioners to understand the possibilities these nurses can offer us now.

NURSING INTERVENTIONS: INFLUENCING CHANGE

Sylvia Rinker explores the meaning of the obstetrical experience and how nurses supported its move to the hospital and a more medical orientation during the first half of the twentieth century. In her chapter, *Obstetric Nursing: For the Patient or the Doctor?*, Rinker questions the current high maternal morbidity rates (15 deaths per 100,000 live births) in the United States (which is higher than 33 other countries) given the high cost and advanced specialization of obstetrical practice in hospital settings. She traces it to the early 1900s when both physicians and newly educated nurses encouraged birthing women to turn away from midwife-attended home births and to enter hospitals for a scientific medical birth experience. From the 1900s to the 1940s, nurses vigilantly maintained asepsis and rigidly applied rules separating mothers from their families during delivery. By the 1940s, however, Rinker writes that nurses who worked in this specialization began to develop and exercise their own expertise in the care of these patients throughout the birthing process. They expanded their role from that of a subordinate to that complementary to physicians. Given the historical evidence, Rinker asks nurses today to consider the power of their role as they try to humanize the birthing experience within a medical environment.

Cancer, the second leading cause of death since 1920, still remains a major health care concern. Brigid Lusk, in *Nursing Patients With Cancer in the 1950s: New Issues and Old Challenges*, reflects on nurses' roles in cancer care during the 1950s as a way to help nurses reclarify what nursing is and what it does. The mid-twentieth century saw the development of new treatments for cancer that required nurses to find innovative ways to support their patients undergoing such treatments. According to Lusk, patients who experienced the newer radical and often disfiguring surgeries, radiation treatments, and anticancer drug therapies of the 1950s required nursing care to help them through the ordeal. Nurses and the interventions they devised in response to newer treatments helped patients achieve some level of well-being and normalcy. Also, concern for safety of both the patient and nurse emerged as radiation therapies became more common. Yet little knowledge about safety-related issues placed nurses and patients at risk during these treatments. Equally troubling for some nurses was the need to support the physician's decision to withhold from patients information about their diagnosis. Examining how nurses cared for patients with cancer during the 1950s shows us the challenges nurses experienced as they adapted to changes in cancer treatments, supported patient well-being, addressed issues of safety, and questioned (or not) the necessity to inform patients of their diagnosis. Studying these historical challenges assists nurses reflect on similar challenges today.

In *Trial and Negotiation in a Technological System: Case Study of the Swan-Ganz Catheter*, Kathleen G. Burke shows how nurses influence the adoption of new technology in practice. In her chapter, Burke uses the introduction and gradual acceptance of the Swan-Ganz catheter, a new technology introduced in the sugical intensive care unit at the Hospital of University of Pennsylvania in the 1960s and 1970s, as an exemplar. Stories of nurses who participated in the introduction of the Swan-Ganz catheter show how they influenced the gradual adoption of this new technology into practice. The SICU nurses were part of health care teams that shared knowledge, skills, and developed trust that were essential factors for the adoption of innovative technology.

Karen Flynn also studies nurses' relationship with technology in her chapter, *Black Canadian Nurses and Technology*, which explores the experience of Black Canadian nurses and their response to the introduction of technology in practice from the 1960s until the 1990s. Flynn adds the perspective of race to the concept of gender as she explores the oral histories of Black nurses, who were educated in Canada, the Caribbean, and Great Britain before immigration to Canada. Including these women's voices in the discussion, Flynn writes from a more theoretical perspective, and adds to the "polyvocality" of perspectives and a broader interpretation of nurses' relationship with technology. The Black Canadian nurses interviewed entered nursing between the 1950s and 1970s and witnessed an explosive increase in the use of medical technology in practice. Yet, their acceptance of technology varied. Their experiences show how current discussions about nurses and technology must take into account the broader social, political, and economic context to better understand the complicated dynamics between nurses and the technologies they use.

NURSING INTERVENTIONS: NEGOTIATING SPACE

Rima D. Apple's chapter, *To Avoid Expense and Suffering: Public Health Nurses and the Struggle for Health Services,* shows the challenges public health nurses experienced as they sought to bring services to rural counties in Wisconsin during the 1940s. Using the Wisconsin Bureau of Maternal Child Health Demonstration Program (MCH) and the example of two MCH nurses, Apple looks at the pivotal role that public health nurses played in assuring communities access to the essential health care they needed. One of the public health nurses, originally hired as part of the demonstration project, was not successful in convincing county board members to hire a permanent public health nurse when the project ended. Her successor, however, did make the case. Although social, economic, and political factors influenced the board's decision, the ability of the MCH nurse to convince them of the efficacy of such a hire was a key nursing intervention. The exemplar Apple presents shows the strategic importance of providing key evidence as nurses advocate for change in health care reform today.

Julie A. Fairman looks at the metaphorical and physical boundaries of the "visit" as the place to explore nurse practitioners' relationships with patients and physicians in her chapter, *The Visit: Nurse Practitioners and the Negotiation of Practice*. Fairman writes about the many factors that shaped nurse practitioners' practice including the context of health care, the place where practice takes place, and the economics of paying for care. She also considers the complex negotiations between and among these various factors, including the boundaries established between the individual nurse practitioner and physician dyad. By returning to the earlier efforts of nurse practitioners to establish their professional identity, nurse practitioners today can better understand the challenges they face in the complex health care setting as they negotiate collaborative agreements. Health care politics, boundary issues, and professional control continue to be part of the negotiations as nurse practitioners provide much-needed health care services to the public.

The need for public policy to support end-of-life care is exemplified in Joy Buck's chapter, *Nursing the Borderlands of Life: Hospice and the Politics of Health Care Reform.* Set in the 1970s, Buck presents nursing's participation in the political struggle to obtain public policies that support hospice services in the United States in hope of understanding the dilemma that Americans face today in obtaining appropriate end-of-life care when needed. Buck uses the historical evidence of the earlier battle to win federal compensation for this care to guide in ways to consider the future battles to come.

Throughout *History as Evidence: Nursing Interventions Through Time,* nurses are seen as negotiating within various political, economic, social, and professional contexts. The skills this negotiation required became part of their nursing interventions. Whether in the hospital or in the home, nurses historically had to find a space they could call their own in which to practice. Nursing interventions have always and still do exist within a larger historical context. From this perspective, the invisibility of nursing's past is now made visible. Our past appears to us anew, sparking new questions about nursing's value and efficacy, then as now.

Section I

NURSING INTERVENTIONS: PROVIDING CARE

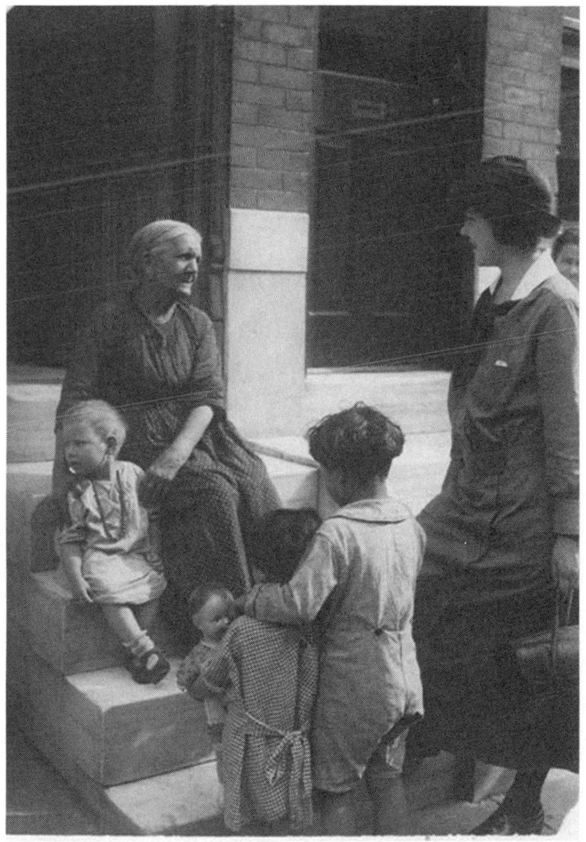

Philadelphia visiting nurse talking with a family, ca. 1925. *Reprinted with permission of the Barbara Bates Center for the Study of the History of Nursing.*

CHAPTER 1

Sweating, Purging, and a Passion for Care: The Yellow Fever Nurse in the Deep South in the Early Nineteenth Century

Linda Sabin

August was hot and steamy in New Orleans in 1853. As the sun rose over the horizon, members of the Howard Association looked forward to another day's events with dread. These volunteer nurses and relief workers had labored in epidemics throughout the region since the 1830s and knew much of what to expect. Yellow fever had come back to the sprawling city on the Mississippi and was feared because of the deadly toll it had taken on the community since its earliest settlement in the previous century. Fever lurked in the climate of the region, and for the new residents and visitors, it could be a deadly visitation. Those who could not flee the city shut themselves up in stifling homes to avoid the deadly air in spite of the soaring temperatures outside. New Orleans residents could look back with horror at the ravages of this disease in previous epidemics and were legitimately fearful of what might unfold.[1]

Black men and women, with their natural resistance to the disease and as survivors of previous outbreaks, would fare better in the days to come because of their immunity to the virus. All those considered immune and willing to

---

[1]Flora Hildreth, "The Howard Association of New Orleans, 1837–1878" (PhD diss., University of California, 1975), 70; Jo Ann Carrigan, *The Saffron Scourge: A History of Yellow Fever in New Orleans* (Lafayette, LA: Center for Louisiana Studies).

give aid would find themselves at the bedside of those struck by the acute fever and would learn nursing by doing what they could in the sickroom. The nursing of the sick would be a makeshift affair, with both the free and enslaved men and women who had not fled helping those in dire need, often with little medical direction. The few physicians who were left had little to offer beyond the harsh laxatives, emetics, blistering, bleeding, cupping, and sweating of patients that were the hallmarks of the medical treatments of the time. Treatment had not changed significantly since the epidemics of the late eighteenth century. In most cases any intervention by either folk remedies or formal medicine were all used in vain to save lives. Many days of watching with a patient and doing all known at the time would still lead to the black vomit then delirium, coma, and death. Fever nursing in the early nineteenth century was dangerous and required enormous energy and stamina.[2]

THE ENVIRONMENT AND THE DISEASE

The environment and the response of the people living in this region set the stage for the disasters that plagued residents. Yellow fever was not the only seasonal plague to affect communities in the Deep South but the frequency of the outbreaks, the disruption of daily life, and the deadliness of the disease caused intense distress in the region. The climate, human behavior, and culture led to a large variety of illnesses. The moist, warm climate with temperate cold seasons stimulated the growth of disease-carrying mosquitoes and waterborne illnesses. The political decision to establish the social and economic system of slavery led to the importation of slaves with an African variant of malaria and yellow fever. These variants combined with local forms of these diseases to make the entire region sickly as seasons waxed and waned. Of all the illnesses of the period, only tuberculosis escaped the restriction of quarantine. Since tuberculosis was viewed as a chronic, wasting disease that attacked susceptible people, it was not viewed as contagious.[3]

---

[2]Erwin Ackerknecht, *Therapeutics from the Primitive to the Twentieth Century* (New York: Hafner Press, 1973), 94–95; William Robinson, *Diary of a Samaritan* (New York: Harper & Brothers, 1860), 44–47, 92–97, 150; Carrigan, *Saffron Scourge*, 30–50.

[3]K. David Patterson, "Disease Environments of the Antebellum South," in *Science and Medicine in the Old South*, eds. Ronald Numbers and Todd Savitt (Baton Rouge, LA: Louisiana State University Press, 1989), 152; James O. Breedon, "Disease as a Factor in Southern Distinctiveness," in *Disease and Distinctiveness in the American South*, eds. Todd L. Savitt and James Harvey Young (Knoxville, TN: University of Tennessee Press, 1989), 1, 2, 9; Lucy Robertson Bridgeforth, "Medicine in Antebellum Mississippi," *Journal of Mississippi* History: 56 (May 1984): 83.

The clinical picture of yellow fever was consistent across all the epidemics in the Deep South. This viral infection began with chills, fever, muscle pains, headache, backache, nausea and vomiting, prostration, and a slow weak pulse. Mild cases resolved in a few days. In more serious cases, the person appeared to be getting better and then collapsed with severe liver disease, jaundice, and hemorrhagic lesions in the stomach and subcutaneous tissues. The classic black vomit indicated deteriorating physical status and what we now know as liver failure.[4] Strategies for addressing yellow fever were empirical: Physicians tried whatever might work and then reported the outcomes of their efforts in the periodical literature of the time.[5] Yellow fever, typhoid, and malaria received the most attention in early Southern medical journals, with the great yellow fever outbreaks stimulating a specialty in that area. Physicians were baffled by the appearance in some years and then apparent absence in others. The miasma theories then current—the idea that emanations from decaying organic matter caused diseases—failed to explain the disease that was ultimately tied to a vector: the mosquito.[6] In addition, the social isolation of much of the region—the agrarian economy, slavery, and chronic poverty that prevailed during this era in much of the Deep South—insulated most communities from innovations and advances in hygiene and sanitation. These community issues shaped the illness experience linked to the outbreaks of yellow fever that raged in most hot seasons.[7]

One formal experience in the early nineteenth-century Deep South was characterized by a small, narrowly focused medical profession that clung to traditional medicine that was known as the "Galenic" approach to healing. This therapeutic system was characterized by the treatment of the four humors

---

[4]David L. Heymann, ed., *Control of Communicable Diseases Manual* (Washington: American Public Health Association, 2008), 684; Carrigan, *Saffron Scourge*, 7–8, 59–60.

[5]George Campbell, "On the Utility of Bloodletting in the Advanced Stages of Fever," *Transylvania Journal of Medicine* 2 (August 1829): 332–343; A. P. Jones, "Yellow Fever in a Rural District," *New Orleans Medical News and Hospital Gazette* 9 (July 1854): 180–209; N. Walkley, "Original Communications: On the Treatment of Yellow Fever, as it Occurred in Mobile in the Fall of 1853," *New Orleans Medical and Surgical Journal* (November 1854): 289–291; John E. Cooke, "On the Use of Cold Water in Fever," *Transylvania Medical Journal* 5 (January 1832): 49–71.

[6]Richard Shryock, "Medical Practice in the Old South," in *Medicine in America: Historical Essays* (Baltimore, MD: Johns Hopkins University Press, 1966), 55; Jo Ann Carrigan, "Yellow Fever: Scourge of the South," in *Disease and Distinctiveness in the American South*, eds. Todd L. Savitt and James Harvey Young (Knoxville, TN: University of Tennessee Press), 55–71.

[7]Carrigan, "Yellow Fever," 69–71; Bridgeforth, "Medicine in Antebellum Mississippi," 104; Martha Carolyn Mitchell, "Health and Medical Practice in the Lower South," *Journal of Southern History*, 10 (November 1944): 432–435.

in the body, blood, yellow bile, black bile, and phlegm, which were considered the source of most imbalances in the body. The treatment for the imbalance can be traced back to Hippocrates and Galen who encouraged aggressive efforts to rid the body of the bad humors. This required purging, blistering, cupping, and bleeding, and all of these treatments depleted the patient of body fluids and/or blood. Benjamin Rush had used copious bleeding, purging, and blistering in his treatment of patients during the severe yellow fever outbreak in Philadelphia in 1797. He wrote about his strategies and they were still taught in medical schools of the time.[8]

One exception to this typically aggressive approach to traditional medicine came from Europe. It was practiced in New Orleans where a large French/Creole medical community offered a different approach to fever care. The French physicians, following the divergent therapies adopted in their homeland, rejected Galen's humors and believed in a milder approach to all the fevers. They favored symptom relief and support of the patient through meticulous nursing care, bland foods, and a mixture of fluids. During this period, the beginnings of other forms of alternative treatments began to receive attention. Homeopathy was a therapy that taught to give medications, diluted many times that were supposed to mimic the symptoms of the fever. Water therapists or hydropaths believed in using just water therapies in fevers. Thomsonists, a botanical, self-help approach that was developed by a northern botanist named Samuel Thomson, believed that herbal cures combined with care from family members, avoidance of alcohol, and repentance of sin would be as effective as traditional medicine.[9]

Nursing was primarily domestic in nature with loved ones, friends, and neighbors helping the afflicted. Domestic nurses at home provided the less visible, home-based bedside care within the family unit at times of need.[10] Some fewer community nurses provided visible, recognized nursing care during periods of crisis or change in a community.[11] Only in the larger communities such as New Orleans, Mobile, and Natchez did relief and nursing care become organized in any way.

Table 1.1 presents examples of common traditional and alternative therapies used during this period. Table 1.2 shows some of the nursing functions carried out during the treatment of patients with fevers.

---

[8]John Duffy, "Medical Practice in the Ante Bellum South," *Journal of Southern History* 25, no. 1 (February 1959): 52–70; Shryock, "Medical Practice in the Old South," 62–63.

[9]Bridgeforth, "Medicine in Antebellum Mississippi," 90–92; Carrigan, *Saffron Scourge*, 315–316; Cooke, "The Use of Cold Water in Fever," 62–69; Duffy, "Medical Practice in the Ante Bellum South," 67–69.

[10]Linda E. Sabin, "From the Home to the Community: A History of Nursing in Mississippi, 1870-1940" (PhD diss., University of Mississippi, 1994), 18.

[11]Ibid., 17.

TABLE 1.1 Common Traditional and Alternative Therapies Used in the Deep South During the Early Nineteenth Century

Symptom	Fever	Nausea/Vomiting/Diarrhea	Malaise/Chills	Pain	Additional Symptoms/ Prostration/Coma
Traditional treatments	Early—vigorous bleeding[a,b] Large doses of quinine until the patient got dizzy or passed out[b,c] Application of cold water either over the head or by soaking[a] Late in the disease sweating is to be induced, more quinine given with opium[d] No food or water until the fever subsides or small amounts of water only[b]	Ipecac to open and drain the stomach[c] Calomel and Jalap (strong mercurial laxatives) to purge the bowels.[b] If purging was not complete, enemas were used with cold water to reduce temperature and open bowels[d] Blisters aspplied to epigastrium to remove humors[d] Stimulating enemas to speed evacuation of the bowels[d]	Warm mustard baths to the feet Keep in bed with multiple covers regardless of room temperature[b,d]	Blister affected area to remove the pain[a,d,e] Provide opium with purging medications[b] Counter irritation: application of hot poultices or counter irritants (substances to inflame the skin) applied to painful areas to draw out pain[b] Cupping with scarification to stimulate blood flow and remove humors from within[d]	Stimulants—usually in the form of alcohol, whiskey, champagne, or brandy[a,d] Warmth—placing the patient under many covers to sweat out the fever[d] Bleeding in large amounts to release the cause of the fever after all other therapies have failed[a]
Supportive French therapies	Sponging with tepid water[b] Warm and cool drinks to patient's preference and tolerance[b]	Emollient enemas[b]	Warm foot baths[b]	Massage, opium per needs[b]	Leeches used for inflammation[b]
Thomsonism	Home care by nurse maintaining normal diet[b,e]	Botanical herbal treatments and fluids[c,e]	Steam baths[c,e]		Abstain from alcohol and let nature take its course[c,b]
Homeopathic treatment	Quinine in minute doses[b]	Ipecac in minute doses[b]	Warmth/ Sweating[d]	Opium in minute doses[b]	General supportive care. All drugs given in minute doses to mimic the symptoms.[b]
Hydropathic treatment—water cure	Ice-cold water in copious amounts[d,e]	Cold water enemas[d,e]	Wet, cold sheets applied and removed[d,e]	Wet packs applied to areas of pain.[e]	

[a]Alexander Biddle, Family Letters (Benjamin Rush), Yellow Fever, 1797, Philadelphia (Philadelphia, PA: J.B. Lippincott, 1892), 10, 15, 21, 24.
[b]Carrigan, The Saffron Scourge: A History of Yellow Fever in Louisiana, 1796–1905, 24–25, 37–38, 68, 294–296, 300, 303, 304, 315, 318.
[c]Duffy, "Medical Practice in the Ante Bellum South," 53–56, 66–71.
[d]Robertson, Diary of a Samaritan, 25, 34–35, 44–47, 92–93, 132–133, 152, 157–158.
[e]Bridgeforth, "Medicine in Antebellum Mississippi," 56, 86–94.

Nursing practice was dictated by the norms for medical practice in the day. The entire region remained rural and isolated with only New Orleans reaching urban status before the Civil War. Epidemics tended to be seasonal and localized to a specific geographical area. It has been noted in recent historical research that all major yellow fever outbreaks in the nineteenth-century South entered the region through New Orleans and became regional by spreading upriver to the inland north of the city.[12]

DOMESTIC AND COMMUNITY NURSES IN THE EARLY NINETEENTH CENTURY

Evidence about nursing during this period is dispersed and fragmented, with nurses only indirectly appearing in the writings of physicians or diarists. In fact, almost all caregivers can be classified as domestic nurses: men and women who cared for loved ones, neighbors, slaves, or friends in time of need. Such nurses often lacked the direction of a physician when providing care. Of course, the majority of citizens in the region then were rural, poorly educated farmers or tradesmen and families. Only in the last several years before the Civil War did a small elite class of planters and entrepreneurs develop along the rivers of the "Black Belt" of the Deep South. We should also recall that the era of the great plantations was short lived, involving a small minority of the population in the region. The men and women who provided the bedside care in times of epidemic fever outbreaks were serving persons who were significant to them.[13] In some early articles in medical journals, pioneer physicians report having to serve as nurse as well as doctor in some cases because entire families were ill and there was of a lack of caregivers.[14]

A small number of community nurses were those who served persons outside of their acquaintance out of charity or for a salary. The actual practice of these nurses was determined by the physicians directing care or by the individual nurse's experience. Certainly, there was little standardization to treatment modalities. Most of the known cures or treatments were found

---

[12]Carrigan, *Saffron Scourge*, 1–4.

[13]Edward Akin, *Mississippi: An Illustrated History* (Northridge, CA: Mississippi Historical Society, 1987), 51.

[14]A. P. Jones, "Yellow Fever in a Rural District," *New Orleans Medical News and Hospital Gazette*, 9 (July 1, 1854): 185; Andrew Kilpatrick, "An Account of Yellow Fever Which Prevailed in Woodville, Mississippi, 1844," *New Orleans Medical Journal* 2 (July 1845): 44–48.

in household manuals and passed from generation to generation by word and example. Local pharmacies and general stores were the primary providers of patent and other medicines for the public during these outbreaks. One survey of sales from this period showed that the most common drugs sold to the general public were quinine, paregoric, castor oil, oil of tartar, alum, Epsom salts, camphor, ipecac, calomel, laudanum, and tincture of opium. In addition to these classic remedies, the sales of whiskey and brandy as stimulants and pain relievers exceeded that of the others. The few patent medicines available at the time were advertized in columns in New Orleans newspapers and small-town weekly publications.[15]

Nurses were expected to remain with the patient at all times and to carry out instructions. A case of yellow fever was treated first with a hot mustard bath especially to the feet. Strong laxatives were given immediately to keep the bowels open. As the temperature rose, the body was rubbed with either cool cloths since ice was scarce in the late-summer yellow fever season or covered with extra blankets in a heated room to sweat the illness. Physicians, when available, might perform blistering that involved placing hot irons on the feet or over the point of pain. Cupping involved placing glass cups that had been heated by burning alcohol in them on the surface of the skin to draw the heat from the body. Cupping might be done by a doctor or in the cities by a "Cupper" who had skill in this procedure. Bleeding was used as an accepted approach to protect the patient from the ravages of yellow fever until the late antebellum period. Lancing a vessel or applying leeches until the patient receiving treatment fainted accomplished bleeding. Sickrooms were hot and stuffy because of the fear of fresh air bringing more infection from the emanations of the outside environment. Nurses were expected to provide the baths, clean up from the purging, and provide friction rubs to stimulate a failing patient or cooling cloths to a delirious patient with a high fever. Fever nurses were exposed to contagion in a variety of ways and risked their own health in the illness environment.[16]

If the nurses followed the alternative approaches that gained favor in the region later in the study period, then there was more watching and waiting as the gentler approaches provided nourishment, physical treatments, and supportive strategies to help the patient handle the illness. While the outcome was still often death of the patient, the stress on both the patient and the caregiver was reduced.

---

[15]Duffy, "Medical Practice in the Ante Bellum South," 64–66; Carrigan, *Saffron Scourge*, 319–322.

[16]Robinson, *Diary of a Samaritan*, 22–26, 44–47, 92–97; Duffy, "Medical Practice in the Ante Bellum South," 66–67; Bridgeforth, "Medicine in Antebellum Mississippi," 86–87.

TABLE 1.2 Functions of Nurses Practicing with Traditional and Alternative Therapies in the Deep South During the Early Nineteenth Century

Medical Treatment/ Medication	Nursing Role in Preparation	Nursing Role in Implementation	Presence Required
Bleeding	Positioning patient in bed, protecting the bed, providing catch basin or bucket[a,b]	Holding patient in position in case of uncooperativeness or painful response[a]	Needed to assist and to help bandage and observe after the procedure. If abortive bleeding is done, patient will bleed until fainting and must be protected until consciousness returns.[a]
Emetics/laxatives	Prepare the powders or liquids or measure the tinctures and create the mixtures for the dosing. Administer medications as ordered or assist doctor in dosing.[a,b,c]	Provide basin or bucket—clean up patient after vomiting and bowel movements[a]	Remain with patient and remove vomitus and excreta.[a]
Enemas/clysters	Mix the enema solutions and prepare the bed to protect from the fluid and excreta. Maintain a smooth pipe on the clyster tube. Position chair and chamber pot or bucket nearby.[a,d]	Administer the enema and help patient position to expel the liquid. Protect the bed.[d]	Remain with the patient until enema is expelled and clean up remains.[a,d]
Cupping and scarification	The "cupper" or physician will prepare the cups[a,b,c]	The nurse will help position and secure the patient who may respond to the pain of the procedure unless extremely depleted.[a]	Comfort care to the cupping area and provision of fluids after the procedure are needed for the patient.[a]
Bathing/sponging	Preparation of the bed for sponging to protect from the water or water and vinegar. Preparation of bathtub if bathing is possible. Position a chair in a tub if patient is to be showered with cold water.[a,b,c]	Encouraging or coaxing an ill fever patient to bathe took skill and the ability to maneuver an often unwilling person into an awkward tub. Sponging was also often met with resistance and uncooperativeness.[a]	Patience and persistence were critical for the fever nurse who might be sponging for hours or providing support for frequent baths or cold water showers each day.[a,d]

Counterirritants, poultices, and fomentations	Each physician or home guide had recipes and instructions on preparation. Commonly used: turpentine rubs, mustard poultices[a,c]	Causing irritation, blisters, and inflammation to the skin with the aim to relieve deep-seated inflammation was a painful process not received well by sick fever patients. Nurses had to use skill and patience when achieving the goal of the therapy.[a]	These treatments often caused infected lesions that had to be observed and cared for. The treatments could create animosity between the nurse and the patient and they were exhausting to provide several times a day.[a]
Massage/heat/cold applications	Preparation of cool cloths, warm packs, or mixture of massage creams or compounds[a,c]	Provide the heat or cold regularly for days when dealing with chills, fever, need to sweat, or relieve pain[a,c]	Comfort measures were often the only strategy that brought sleep or rest for an exhausted fever patient. These measures were needed day and night. When chill was feared or they were sweating the illness, all applications were done with the covers on the patient.[a,c]
Diet considerations	Preparation of sickroom meals was time consuming—beef tea, barley and rice water, and even securing ice or cool water involved time and effort.	Helping fever patients take nourishment in small quantities around the clock was a major function for bedside nurses. Often intake was restricted to small amounts every few minutes in an effort to keep fluids down.	This function was often frustrating for nurses since patients who had been vigorously purged, vomited quite easily.[a]
	Withholding food and fluid was often the order for the patient[a,c]	Refusing a patient fluids and food could be time consuming and frustrating.[a]	
End-of-life care	Care of the patient who is dying[a]	Relating the needs of the patient to the family and doctor if one is available[a]	Being with the patient in the room or home during the dying process[a,b]

Note: Many of these activities appear in William Robinson's diary or are implied in the treatment articles in Table 1.1, some of these descriptions come from relating the tasks that would flow from the Galenic and alternative therapies given that the nurse would be the only other person in the room with the physician or perhaps being the person who actually provided the therapies. The presence in the room created need for the nurse to perform these tasks that were created by the treatments. Included in all of the tasks of the nurse was the presence, watching, waiting, and responding to the changing condition of the patient.

[a]Robinson, *Diary of a Samaritan,* 16, 22–26, 35–36, 40–47, 56–59, 62–63, 92–97, 141, 171–177, 182.

[b]Carrigan, *Saffron Scourge*, 11, 68, 292.

[c]Kilpatrick, "An Account of Yellow Fever," 44–48.

[d]Johnson, *Friendly Cautions to Families and Others*, 155–159.

DOMESTIC NURSES

During this era, and particularly on plantations and larger farms, white and black women and some black men performed domestic nursing practice. Extensive research in the history of Southern women documented the role of plantation mistresses and selected female slaves in the care of sick slaves.[17] The women from both races served the needs of slaves suffering from local outbreaks of yellow fever. Meeting the daily needs of patients suffering the symptoms of yellow fever became the duty of those nearest the patient. All household servants regardless of race might be pressed into service when an epidemic raged.

Black women, in their role as slaves, made a major contribution to domestic nursing during the early nineteenth century. They cared for their own families using the remedies passed down within their community. They also contributed to the care of white families in the homes where they acted as enslaved servants. It must be noted that this role did not end with [illegible] but endured to the mid-twentieth century.[19] It was assumed that these wo[illegible] would serve any family member in times of illness. This combined wi[illegible] natural immunity to yellow fever made African American women [illegible] preferred nurses during outbreaks.[20]

Grandma Venus, the only name by which we know her, was a re[illegible] nurse in the antebellum home of the pioneer Sharkey family in Mi[illegible] Grandma Venus had grown up with Clay Sharkey's mother and [illegible] her by her father when she married. She cared the children and [illegible] family through two generations of Sharkeys. Clay Sharkey wrote [illegible] great affection, remembering her care in times of sickness and [illegible] that Grandma Venus stayed with the family even after emancipa[illegible]

---

[17]Todd L. Savitt, "Slave Health and Medical Distinctiveness," in Disease [illegible] the American South, 142–143; Catherine Clinton, The Plantation Mistress [illegible] University Press, 1982), 145; Elizabeth Fox-Genovese, Within the Plantatio[illegible] White Women of the Old South (Charlotte, NC: University of North Caro[illegible]

[18]Susan Tucker, Telling Memories Among Southern Women: Dom[illegible] Employers in the Segregated South (New York: Schocken Books, 198[illegible]

[19]Fox-Genovese, Within the Plantation Household, 291; Jennie W[illegible] with Mrs. D. W. Giles, in The American Slave: A Composite Biogr[illegible] Supplemental Series 10 (Westport, CT: Greenwood Press, [illegible] Health and Medical Distinctiveness," 124, 145–146. This [illegible] nations for the immunity of African Americans to yellow fever [illegible]

[20]George Osborne, "Plantation Life in Central Mississippi as [illegible] Papers," Journal of Mississippi History 3 (November 1941): 2[illegible]

Counterirritants, poultices, and fomentations	Each physician or home guide had recipes and instructions on preparation. Commonly used: turpentine rubs, mustard poultices[a,c]	Causing irritation, blisters, and inflammation to the skin with the aim to relieve deep-seated inflammation was a painful process not received well by sick fever patients. Nurses had to use skill and patience when achieving the goal of the therapy.[a]	These treatments often caused infected lesions that had to be observed and cared for. The treatments could create animosity between the nurse and the patient and they were exhausting to provide several times a day.[a]
Massage/heat/cold applications	Preparation of cool cloths, warm packs, or mixture of massage creams or compounds[a,c]	Provide the heat or cold regularly for days when dealing with chills, fever, need to sweat, or relieve pain[a,c]	Comfort measures were often the only strategy that brought sleep or rest for an exhausted fever patient. These measures were needed day and night. When chill was feared or they were sweating the illness, all applications were done with the covers on the patient.[a,c]
Diet considerations	Preparation of sickroom meals was time consuming—beef tea, barley and rice water, and even securing ice or cool water involved time and effort.	Helping fever patients take nourishment in small quantities around the clock was a major function for bedside nurses. Often intake was restricted to small amounts every few minutes in an effort to keep fluids down.	This function was often frustrating for nurses since patients who had been vigorously purged, vomited quite easily.[a]
	Withholding food and fluid was often the order for the patient[a,c]	Refusing a patient fluids and food could be time consuming and frustrating.[a]	
End-of-life care	Care of the patient who is dying[a]	Relating the needs of the patient to the family and doctor if one is available[a]	Being with the patient in the room or home during the dying process[a,b]

Note: Many of these activities appear in William Robinson's diary or are implied in the treatment articles in Table 1.1, some of these descriptions come from relating the tasks that would flow from the Galenic and alternative therapies given that the nurse would be the only other person in the room with the physician or perhaps being the person who actually provided the therapies. The presence in the room created need for the nurse to perform these tasks that were created by the treatments. Included in all of the tasks of the nurse was the presence, watching, waiting, and responding to the changing condition of the patient.

[a]Robinson, *Diary of a Samaritan*, 16, 22–26, 35–36, 40–47, 56–59, 62–63, 92–97, 141, 171–177, 182.

[b]Carrigan, *Saffron Scourge*, 11, 68, 292.

[c]Kilpatrick, "An Account of Yellow Fever," 44–48.

[d]Johnson, *Friendly Cautions to Families and Others*, 155–159.

DOMESTIC NURSES

During this era, and particularly on plantations and larger farms, white and black women and some black men performed domestic nursing practice. Extensive research in the history of Southern women documented the role of plantation mistresses and selected female slaves in the care of sick slaves.[17] The women from both races served the needs of slaves suffering from local outbreaks of yellow fever. Meeting the daily needs of patients suffering the symptoms of yellow fever became the duty of those nearest the patient. All household servants regardless of race might be pressed into service when an epidemic raged.

Black women, in their role as slaves, made a major contribution to domestic nursing during the early nineteenth century. They cared for their own families using the remedies passed down within their community. They also contributed to the care of white families in the homes where they acted as enslaved servants. It must be noted that this role did not end with slavery but endured to the mid-twentieth century.[18] It was assumed that these women would serve any family member in times of illness. This combined with the natural immunity to yellow fever made African American men and women preferred nurses during outbreaks.[19]

Grandma Venus, the only name by which we know her, was a respected nurse in the antebellum home of the pioneer Sharkey family in Mississippi. Grandma Venus had grown up with Clay Sharkey's mother and was given to her by her father when she married. She reared the children and nursed the family through two generations of Sharkeys. Clay Sharkey wrote of her with great affection, remembering her care in times of sickness and was grateful that Grandma Venus stayed with the family even after emancipation.[20]

---

[17]Todd L. Savitt, "Slave Health and Medical Distinctiveness," in *Disease and Distinctiveness in the American South*, 142–143; Catherine Clinton, *The Plantation Mistress* (New York: Oxford University Press, 1981), 145; Elizabeth Fox-Genovese, *Within the Plantation Household: Black and White Women of the Old South* (Charlotte, NC: University of North Carolina Press, 1990), 129.

[18]Susan Tucker, *Telling Memories Among Southern Women: Domestic Workers and Their Employers in the Segregated South* (New York: Schocken Books, 1988), 13–17.

[19]Fox-Genovese, *Within the Plantation Household*, 291; Jennie Webb (ex-slave), interview with Mrs. D. W. Giles, in *The American Slave a Composite Biography*, ed. George Rawick, Supplemental Series 10 (Westport, CT: Greenwood Press, 1977), 2250; Savitt, "Slave Health and Medical Distinctiveness," 124, 145–149. This source has one of the best explanations for the immunity of African Americans to yellow fever in the nineteenth century.

[20]George Osborne, "Plantation Life in Central Mississippi, as Revealed in the Clay Sharkey Papers," *Journal of Mississippi History* 3 (November 1941): 280.

COMMUNITY NURSES

Few details remain about some of the earliest epidemics in the region, although there are records of outbreaks of yellow fever in New Orleans in 1796 and Natchez in 1818. Records of physicians' efforts to determine the cause of fever and to eradicate it exist, but the records are silent on the caregivers.[21] The remaining records of community nurses are fragmentary and depict contributions of men as well as women who remained in fever-stricken communities after most of the women and children had been evacuated to rural locations. Men by virtue of staying behind to maintain businesses or secure family property became caregivers once the epidemic took hold and isolated the community.[22]

In 1822, for example, John Estey related his experiences during a vicious outbreak of yellow fever in Port Gibson, Mississippi. First, he wrote to his brother about helping others in the epidemic since one of his friends had died: He felt he had to do something to help the sick. The next month he wrote to his mother and sister of a woman he referred to as Aunt Coty who served the entire community throughout the epidemic and helped those trying to volunteer. Aunt Coty was an emancipated slave who remained in the community after others fled in panic and cared for many newly arrived, unacclimated young men in the town. In his letter to his family, he shared how she had worked day and night caring for all of the men's needs. He also described how lonely and fearful the young men were as they suffered with the fever and what a difference she made to their survival.[23]

In the 1830s a voluntary group known as the Howard Association was organized in New Orleans in order to provide community service during epidemics. The practice of immune residents nursing stricken residents as domestic nurses had been a practice before the epidemic of 1837, but the city had grown and needed outstripped available domestic nurses. The Young Men's Howard Association of New Orleans met for the first time on September 15, 1837. The men were from varying socioeconomic classes, with original membership made up of clerks, saddlers, and upper class men living with families and not listed with an occupation; but they did limit the membership to 30 rising young men in the city. The men of the Howard Association served as volunteer nurses and

---

[21]Carrigan, *Saffron Scourge*, 33–54.

[22]Linda Sabin, "Unheralded Nurses: Male Care Givers in the Nineteenth Century South," *Nursing History Review* 5 (1997): 131–148.

[23]John Estey Papers, Letter to his brother dated 19 October 1822; Letter to his mother and sister Sally, dated 7 November 1822, from Choctaw Agency, Near Monroe County, Mississippi Department of Archives and History, Jackson; Sabin, "Unheralded Nurses," 135.

relief organizers wherever needed in the city. During the first fever epidemic, they served 1,500 people. They divided the city into sections and published their home addresses so that the needy could seek help directly, and they set up slates in local stores where the needy could leave messages. They were nonsectarian and cared for all indigent patients regardless of color, race, or sex. They registered all cases and worked together to see that none were missed. Most of the men, known as "the Howards," gave bedside care with a few acting as coordinators and fundraisers.[24] William Robinson in the *Diary of a Samaritan* recorded many of the activities of this group. In this work, he describes the stress his organization placed on stringent, faithful nursing attention at the bedside and the group's skepticism about the reliance of physicians on their treatments including quinine. He gives a view of practice given by experienced men and women who understood the importance of competent nursing care.

Robinson also writes about how, in 1839, a group of 10 Howards with several female nurses went to Mobile, where the fever was raging and provided door-to-door help for the poorest in that community. Robinson's writings provide a valuable view of the bedside practice of community nurses in this period. This forward-thinking organization utilized immune and experienced nurses regardless of race to meet community needs. His recollections stress the need for vigilance when dealing with fever victims who could seem to improve with quinine and then relapse or who would want more food than their bodies could handle. The clinical practice he described focused on providing the patient with proper food for the disease, comfort, medicines used sparingly, if at all, and meeting the daily needs of the families involved.[25]

In 1839, a serious yellow fever outbreak occurred in New Iberia, Louisiana, and almost every resident who had not evacuated became ill with the virus. The death rate from the fever rose daily and people fled in panic. One woman, known to us only as Felicitè, a free woman of color from Santo Domingo, stayed to nurse the victims. She had experience in caring for victims of yellow fever in her homeland and she nursed the sick, prepared the dead for burial, and supervised funerals for proper care of the victims. She was an older woman and small in stature. She became known as Aunt Felicitè after this disaster—one that killed half the people left in the town. When she died in 1852, the town closed all businesses and schools so everyone would be free to attend the funeral.[26]

---

[24]Hildreth, "Howard Association," 50–51.

[25]Robinson, *Diary of a Samaritan*, 16–23.

[26]William Henry Perrin, *Southwest Louisiana Biographical and Historical Record* (New Orleans, LA: The Gulf Publishing, 1891), 108–109.

In 1843, yellow fever broke out in Rodney, Mississippi, along the Mississippi River. The residents fled from town with the exception of a few men and the victims who were already ill. John McGinly led the men left behind in caring for those stricken with the fever. McGinly had nursed before and taught his peers how to care for victims of the fever. He organized those who could care for others and led the relief efforts until he became ill. This frightened many of the people left in the town and more abandoned the sick. His friend Horace Fulkerson cared for John during his illness and then got sick himself. At this point, their mutual friend John Coleman came to their aid and helped both patients until they were recovered.[27]

By the 1850s, communities in the region had developed enough experience with the fever that organized responses were more common in providing nursing care. The Howards grew in number and expanded their philosophy to several branch organizations throughout the South. During the 1853 epidemic, Natchez and Vicksburg, two of Mississippi's larger river cities, had charity boards sponsored by local religious and business leaders that organized and served during epidemics. Fashioned after the Howards, these groups gave care and raised money to hire community nurses to care for the sick. Natchez leaders agreed to pay a princely sum of three dollars a day for nurses to care for victims. The quality of the nurses varied greatly, but during this epidemic, the value of good nursing was gaining recognition.[28]

The Howards of New Orleans sent relief directly to Jackson, Mississippi, and established a branch in that city during the 1853 outbreak. The Howard Association hired Lucy Tapley, one of the few free women of color in the city at that time, to care for yellow fever victims. Tapley's services in that epidemic earned her a strong reputation as an excellent nurse, and she served many families in the city, including a governor, during her long career. Her competence received notice more than a generation later in a front-page obituary in Jackson.[29]

Three religious orders of women also served in the greater New Orleans area in the early nineteenth century. The Ursulines, a French order arrived in the city in 1725 to oversee a military hospital and cared for patients for 40 years. They then opened an orphanage and started a school. They opened their institutions to care for yellow fever victims in many of the epidemics in the city. The Daughters of Charity of St. Vincent DePaul arrived in New

---

[27]Sabin, "Unheralded Nurses," 137–138.
[28]Works Progress Administration, Record Group 60, vol. 223, History of Adams County, Mississippi Department of Archives and History, Jackson.
[29]Clarion Ledger (Jackson), November 16, 1893.

Orleans in 1830 and took over the management of Charity Hospital in 1834. They took charge of relief efforts in the hospital during the early nineteenth-century epidemics. They also worked with the Howard Association in caring for the sickest patients with the resources they had. Henriette Dilille and Juliette Gaudin, two free women of color who sought to educate children of color, organized the Sisters of the Holy Family order in 1842. During yellow fever epidemics, these women opened their school to care for the slaves and people of color. They also went out to neighboring plantations to help with the sick needing care during epidemics of yellow fever.[30]

CONCLUSION

The nurses of the antebellum period had to overcome fear of contagion and the stress of coping with severely ill people in unsavory and dangerous environments. Even when one could claim immunity to yellow fever, the presence of other forms of fever, which were often overlooked in epidemics, made answering the call to serve a dangerous decision. These nurses cared for loved ones, family, and extended family, or they left their homes and cared for their communities during a time of death and fear. Nurses practiced in the shadows in the early part of the nineteenth century and gradually developed a reputation for making a difference in the survival of this disease long before its prevention was identified. The competence of the Howards and their experienced nurses laid a foundation for physician respect and recognition that would carry into the later nineteenth century. Fever nurses earned a place in the community response to yellow fever in these early years of the century. Their work was hard and filled with risk but they endured, and all that they accomplished make a fascinating saga that provides each new generation of nurses with role models for our own epidemics of unmanageable diseases evolving today.

---

[30]Mary Gehman, *Women and New Orleans: A History* (New Orleans, LA: Margaret Media, 1988), 18–21.

CHAPTER 2

Determining Children's "Best Interests" in the Midst of an Epidemic: A Cautionary Tale From History

Cynthia Anne Connolly

INTRODUCTION

Throughout the first decade of the twenty-first century, the growing awareness of what became known as an "epidemic" of childhood obesity has drawn scrutiny from health care providers, public health officials, and policymakers. Researchers, among them many nurses, documented the multifaceted nature of the problem, including childhood obesity's escalating prevalence; disparities according to race and ethnicity; and the interplay between the complex biological, social, and cultural variables believed to promote or inhibit the condition. Drawing on this scholarship, nurses and other clinicians derived a plethora of approaches to the problem.[1]

---

[1]Bobbie Berkowitz and Marleyse, "Advocating for the Prevention of Childhood Obesity: A Call to Action for Nursing," *The Online Journal of Issues in Nursing* 14 (2009), www.nursingworld.org/MainMenuCategories/ANAMarketplace/ANAPeriodicals/OJIN/TableofContents/Vol142009/No1Jan09/Prevention-of-Childhood-Obesity.aspx (accessed September 23, 2009); Kathryn Smith, "Childhood Obesity: Nursing Policy Implications," *Journal of Pediatric Nursing* 21 (August 2006): 308–310; *Childhood Obesity* (Atlanta, GA: U.S. Department of Health and Human Services, Centers for Disease Control and Prevention, 2009), http://www.cdc.gov/HealthyYouth/obesity/index.htm (accessed September 1, 2009).

Through their participation in contemporary debates surrounding how best to address childhood obesity today, nurses, physicians, and other health care providers unwittingly find themselves in the crosshairs of terrain that has historically been highly contested in the United States: In the middle of a perceived epidemic affecting large numbers of children, especially a condition for which there is no cure, how do health care providers draw on sometimes conflicting data to craft interventions for children? And how does society ultimately decide what specific policies and actions are "in the best interest of the child"? The case study presented in this chapter makes no pretensions to having a solution to this ongoing debate. Rather, it aims to analyze nursing's responses to an earlier public health crisis involving children. Specifically, it traces nurses' embrace of a long-forgotten institution, the preventorium, a facility designed to prevent active disease in tuberculosis (TB)-infected children. The hope is that considering the problems and possibilities inherent in this example, we can see not just the enduring nature of issues surrounding children and their health in the United States but also the complexities nurses face in determining "evidence-based practice" without the benefit of hindsight.

THE "WHITE PLAGUE": AN EARLY TWENTIETH-CENTURY PUBLIC HEALTH CRISIS

As the nation's most visible infectious disease in the early twentieth-century pre-antibiotic era, TB was a national preoccupation. Until streptomycin arrived in the 1940s, no cure for TB existed. In urban areas, the infection caused up to 15% of all deaths, more than any other infectious disease. However, although large numbers of people died from the disease, many more experienced long periods of TB-related debilitation. Minimizing TB's toll on society became the focus of numerous public and private endeavors to address the epidemic known as "The White Plague."[2]

Throughout the first three-quarters of the nineteenth century, TB, like most diseases, was postulated to be hereditary and noncontagious. Physicians as well as the lay public believed that constitutional endowments, hereditarily

---

[2]Mark Caldwell, *The Last Crusade: The War on Consumption 1862–1954* (New York: Atheneum, 1988).

transmitted, promoted or resisted illness. Many also thought that immorality and a "bad" lifestyle resulted in poverty and illness.[3] Notions of TB were radically changed in the 1880s by a new framework through which disease and illness came to be understood.[4] But while German scientist Robert Koch's 1882 isolation of the tubercle bacillus facilitated the emergence of the germ theory, many scientists and clinicians did not immediately discard earlier philosophies. Instead, these older ideas were accommodated, and in many instances incorporated, into newer infectious disease explanatory models.[5] For example, many health care providers continued to imbue racial, ethnic, and socioeconomic variations in TB's incidence as evidence that certain groups needed moral, not just material, uplift.

The first years of the twentieth century, the period of time during which the germ theory's acceptance evolved and public health officials feared that the TB epidemic might spiral out of control, were tumultuous ones in the United States. As the pace of industrialization accelerated, many North Americans moved to urban areas seeking greater opportunities. In addition, waves of immigrants, many of them indigent, poured into the cities of the United States. People crowded into tenements, were often unable to speak English, and frequently engaged in cultural practices foreign to earlier arrivals and the native born. Poverty, inadequate sanitation, crime, and infectious diseases, especially TB, became rampant in the poorer districts.

Moreover, although the germ theory enriched scientists' and society's understanding of TB and spurred the creation of voluntary organizations aimed at fighting the infection, such as the National Tuberculosis Association, it added no effective tools to the curative arsenal. Treatment in the early twentieth century, whether in the home or sanatorium, remained much the same as in the nineteenth century. Adjusting patients' environment, nutrition, and their exercise-to-rest ratio remained therapeutic mainstays along with providing health advice and encouraging the modification of deleterious behaviors.[6]

---

[3]Rene and Jean Dubos, *The White Plague: Tuberculosis, Man, and Society* (New Brunswick, NJ: Rutgers University Press, 1952), 3–11.

[4]Charles E. Rosenberg, "The Bitter Fruit: Heredity, Disease, and Social Thought in Nineteenth Century America," in *From Consumption to Tuberculosis: A Documentary History*, ed. Barbara G. Rosenkrantz (New York: Garland, 1994), 154–194.

[5]Nancy J. Tomes, "American Attitudes Toward the Germ Theory of Disease: Phyllis Allen Richmond Revisited," *Journal of the History of Medicine and Allied Sciences* 52 (January 1997): 17–50.

[6]Barbara Bates, *Bargaining for Life: A Social History of Tuberculosis, 1876–1938* (Philadelphia, PA: University of Pennsylvania Press, 1992), 25–41.

THE 1908 SIXTH INTERNATIONAL CONGRESS ON TUBERCULOSIS

It was at this social and scientific juncture that the United States prepared to host the 1908 Sixth International Congress on tuberculosis. In the past, the Congresses convened in major European cities such as Paris and Berlin. As such, anointing the United States' capital of Washington, DC, as the site for 1908 meant that the world scientific community acknowledged that American science mattered in the fight against TB. For almost a week, hundreds of Congress attendees from Europe, Japan, Canada, and Central and South America joined their hosts in contemplating the latest information related to TB's biological, economic, and social consequences.When not in session, Americans feted their colleagues from abroad at receptions and proudly ushered them on tours of hospitals, clinics, sanatoria, and other TB-related institutions. Newspapers in major cities provided detailed coverage of events and President Theodore Roosevelt gave a rousing speech.[7]

The state of the science for the disease once known as consumption unfurled at the Congress. One of most important issues that attracted much scientific attention focused on the fact that many people infected with the tubercle bacillus did not become ill, while others either recovered or died. A major conference theme centered around the importance of unraveling the intricate interplay between bacteria, host, and environment that appeared to influence the outcome of infection. The 80 American nurses in attendance at the Congress recognized the importance of this issue. They arrived brimming with confidence—and armed with data—designed to convince physicians, policy makers, and the public that nurses' role in preventing infection from progressing to illness was a critical one. Nurses' participation in the Congress represented an important milestone for their new profession. Although nursing leaders had been formally meeting since the 1890s when they created the American Society of Superintendents of Training Schools for Nurses (1893) and the Nurses' Associated Alumnae (1896), they surely knew that this meeting was different. For the first time,

---

[7]Theodore Roosevelt, quoted in *Sixth International Congress on Tuberculosis*, vol. 5 (Philadelphia, PA: William F. Fell, 1908), 67–68; "Here to Study War on Tuberculosis," *New York Times*, September 24, 1908, 9; "Seek Method in Germ War: Angelenos to Attend Congress of Tuberculosis," *Los Angeles Times*, September 13, 1908, II3; "Plan War on Tuberculosis: Delegates Flock to Washington," *Boston Daily Globe*, September 14, 1908, 12; "Impetus to War on Tuberculosis: Official Opening of World Congress on White Plague Set for Today," *Chicago Daily Tribune*, September 28, 1909, 12.

American nurses as a group would visibly bring their expertise to bear at an interdisciplinary, international convention focused on a critically important *clinical* problem.[8]

While poverty-related conditions such as an inadequate living environment, excessive crowding, overwork, and insufficient nutrition clearly enhanced one's risk for developing TB, these social problems were, by themselves, too nonspecific to categorize as predisposing criteria unique to TB. Epidemiological investigations revealed that accepting personal responsibility for one's health, practicing good hygiene, and taking regular exercise, for example, all played a role in disease progression, though researchers often disagreed with one another on the extent of each individual variable's influence.

There was, however, consensus on the importance of focusing attention on the pediatric patient. Attendees were excited by the work presented during the Congress's pediatric sessions. Just a few years earlier, a scientific finding had shocked the anti-TB community. Until 1903, many believed that children between the ages of 5 and 15 years possessed special resistance to TB because there were fewer TB-related pediatric than adult deaths. But several early twentieth-century researchers demonstrated that many children who died from non–TB related causes (e.g., such as accidents) harbored the tubercle bacillus.[9] But before the 1908 Congress, postmortem examination remained the only way to identify infected children who lacked recognizable symptoms of disease.

The discovery by Austrian physician Clemens von Pirquet, presented at the Congress, energized Congress attendees because it offered the possibility of identifying "pretubercular" children. Pirquet argued that a byproduct of tubercle bacilli culture, known as tuberculin, could be used to identify those individuals who were infected with TB before they developed actual symptoms. According to his theory, which was quickly accepted by the scientific community, redness and swelling after the injection of a small amount of tuberculin under the skin revealed exposure to the bacillus.[10]

Before tuberculin, clinicians classified children into two groups with regard to TB, the sick and the well. After 1908, a third disease category was

---

[8]L. L. Dock, "The International Congress on Tuberculosis in Washington," *American Journal of Nursing* 9 (November 1908): 93–97.
[9]Maurice Fishberg, *Pulmonary Tuberculosis*, 2nd ed. (Philadelphia, PA: Lea & Feabiger, 1919).
[10]Clemens von Pirquet, "Frequency of Tuberculosis in Childhood," *Journal of the American Medical Association* 52 (February 1909): 675–679.

created, pre-TB. Pretubercular children comprised those infected with the organism, but without active disease. Pirquet's work meshed with the theme of the Congress's pediatric section; the pediatric papers contained similar thematic elements, no matter what aspect of TB they addressed. Presenters almost universally agreed that the incidence of active disease in poor children could be reduced by a series of concrete interventions, including aggressive screening using tuberculin, better hygiene, improved nutrition, ample fresh air, and child and parental education for those youngsters considered most at risk for TB.

Speakers exhorted one another to return home and put TB prevention in children at the center of their anti-TB programs.[11] Resolutions passed at the end of the Congress document that this meeting helped refocus the direction of the TB movement away from treatment of adults toward prevention in children. Moreover, the conference generated a momentum that paved the way for the development of regional TB organizations, groups that spearheaded state and local legislation and worked closely with health departments and schools. Imprinted on delegates' minds was the health education, case finding, and other central public health roles that nurses claimed for themselves at the Congress's nursing sessions, which were packed to capacity with other nurses, physicians, public health officials, legislators, and the leadership of the National Tuberculosis Association.[12]

NURSES AND THE PREVENTORIUM

Seizing upon the new tuberculin test, the public health community sought to use it as an efficient tool to identify pretubercular children. One idea that attracted publicity was the notion of sending them to a brand new type of institution, a "preventorium." This facility seemed to represent the most efficacious strategy to minimize the potential for a TB-infected child to progress to one sick with active TB. The first preventorium was founded in 1909 in the New Jersey town of Lakewood (it soon moved to Farmingdale) with the aim of preventing TB in indigent New York City children, the nation's largest metropolis. Children at the preventorium received therapies considered the cornerstone of TB prevention and treatment during this era. They spent as much time as

---

[11] *Transactions of the Sixth International Congress on Tuberculosis*, vol. 2, section IV, 355–711.
[12] James A. Miller, "Beginnings of the Antituberculosis Movement," *American Review of Tuberculosis* 48 (June 1943): 367; Bates, *Bargaining for Life*, 128.

possible out of doors in camplike settings where they received their education, meals, and rest.

Within a few years, cities and towns around the nation began fundraising for their own preventorium. The campaign to institutionalize poor children suspected to be at high risk for developing TB expanded after World War I. A media barrage in the professional literature and the lay press helped popularize the movement. By the early 1930s, dozens, perhaps hundreds, of such institutions operated throughout the United States, all modeled on the one at Farmindale.[13] Some operated as private, voluntary institutions similar to Farmindale, while others were founded with private funds but managed by public agencies such as public health departments or school districts. Still others functioned in conjunction with public or private hospitals or sanatoria. Unlike Farmindale, however, many preventoria restricted admission by sex, ethnicity, religion, or race. Despite the fact that TB morbidity and mortality was much higher in African American children, for example, there were no institutions in the South in which they were welcome, and few in the Northern states. In other words, preventoria were organized to function around the idiosyncrasies of individual communities, not epidemiological evidence revealing which children were most at risk.[14]

The preventorium idea embodied the leading edge of not just one popular reform movement, but two: TB prevention and "child saving." Children represented a powerful unifying force during this era; those who disagreed with one another on debates roiling the country, such as whether immigration was altering national character, and if so, whether the change was for better or worse, could almost always agree that children were "innocent" and, as such, deserved an investment in their health and social welfare.

Reformers of the late nineteenth and early twentieth century, a period of societal restructuring remembered today as the Progressive Era, believed that aiding children benefited all of American society. Improving the lot of the children of the poor and working classes through measures to promote health and minimize morbidity and mortality, prevent child labor and abuse, and mandate school attendance, for example, were so integral to the Progressive mission of societal uplift that many reformers referred to themselves simply as "child-savers."[15]

---

[13]Cynthia A. Connolly, *Saving Sickly Children: The Tuberculosis Preventorium in American Life, 1909–1970* (New Brunswick, NJ: Rutgers University Press, 2008).

[14]*A Directory of Sanitoria, Hospitals, Day Camps and Preventoria for the Treatment of Tuberculosis in the United States* (New York: NTA, 1923).

[15]Michael B. Katz, *In the Shadow of the Poorhouse: A Social History of Welfare in the United States* (New York: Basic Books, 1986).

In order to have their health "saved" at preventoria, children resided for months, sometimes years, at the institutions. Building on the major role nurses carved out for themselves at the 1908 TB Congress, preventoria were often founded and almost always managed by nurses and there was broad support among nurses for the idea. Meeting each year at the annual National Tuberculosis Association conferences, nurses shared their preventorium-related work with one another. Speaking to her colleagues at the nineteenth annual National Tuberculosis Association meeting in 1923, for example, Colorado public health nurse Ida Spaeth stressed the nurse's role:

> The service the public health nurse can render the preventorium and the tuberculous child is invaluable. She is the connecting link between the home and the institution; between the child and his physician; between the public and the tuberculous child in need of preventorium care. Whether she works out from the institution or in the community as the public health nurse, her responsibility and opportunity toward the tuberculous child and the preventorium are alike. . . .[16]

Physicians, nurses, and others assumed that middle- and upper-class families had the resources and knowledge to provide a healthy atmosphere for their children. TB's ongoing conflation with immorality, poverty, and "bad" living, however, resulted in a belief that poor children required more than therapeutics such as sunlight (heliotherapy), good food, and rest. They also thought that these youngsters needed exposure to the social conditions and moral climate of the wealthier classes, treatment that was to be supplied through institution's nurses.

Jessie Palmer Quimby was one such nurse. As a registered nurse at the Farmingdale Tuberculosis Preventorium for Children in rural New Jersey for more than 30 years, from 1909 until the late 1930s, Quimby was one of the nation's premier preventorium nurses. Since the preventorium strove to be a health care facility, she needed to be available 24 hours a day, so she lived there. Although one could argue that this limited her prospects for a well-rounded life, her professional entrepreneurialism allowed her to forge a unique and powerful role for herself, given the importance society placed on child saving and TB prevention. Farmingdale's physician-in-chief Alfred F. Hess charged Quimby with monitoring the children's physical health, observing them for

---

[16]Ida Spaeth, "The Public Health Nurse, the Tuberculosis Problem and the Child in the Sanatorium," *Transactions of the National Tuberculosis Association* 19 (1923): 438–439.

illness, educating them about hygiene, and supervising all aspects of life at the institution "from the day she fetches them from the railroad station until she returns them to their families."[17]

Upon the arrival of each child, Quimby performed an initial health assessment and weighed him or her. New admissions spent their first 2 weeks isolated from the other children in the quarantine building in an effort to minimize the regular outbreaks of measles, chickenpox, or other communicable diseases.[18] During this time, Quimby got to know the patients, making general estimations of the individual child's health and symptomatology.[19] Since Quimby oversaw every aspect of the children's strict schedule, it became her timetable as well. At the end of the quarantine period, the children moved to their assigned cottages, where the schedule deviated little from day to day. Just like other institutionalized children during this era, preventorium children awoke to a bell, bathed, and proceeded immediately to breakfast. The rest of the day was spent following a structured timetable that included four more meals, play, lessons at the open-air school, rest, and instruction in sewing or housework for girls and mechanics and industrial training for boys. Education on personal hygiene and healthy living, with specific guidelines dictated according to Hess's, Quimby's, and the board of directors' beliefs completed the institution's set of rules. The bedtime of 6:30 P.M. in the winter and 7:30 P.M. in the summer was strictly enforced and children slept dormitory style on the porch, even in the blowing snow of a New Jersey winter.

In addition to her role monitoring children's physical well-being, Quimby disciplined them when they misbehaved. A central nursing task included creating and maintaining an environment superior to that of the child's home. Since overseeing the daily operations of the institution consumed Quimby's days, she must have been exhausted when a sick child kept her on duty into the night. As a result of these daunting responsibilities, her time was almost as structured as that of her young patients. Indeed, Quimby's work kept her so busy that she even had her family

---

[17]"Organizational Report of the First Preventorium in the United States," November 9, 1909, Nathan Straus papers, box 8, Humanities and Social Sciences Library, Manuscripts and Archives Division, New York Public Library; First Medical Report of the Preventorium, July to November 1909, Nathan Straus papers, box 8, Humanities and Social Sciences Library, Manuscripts and Archives Division, New York Public Library.

[18]Farmingdale Annual Report, 1926, National Library of Medicine, Bethesda, Maryland.

[19]Farmingdale Annual Report, 1927–1928, New York Historical Society.

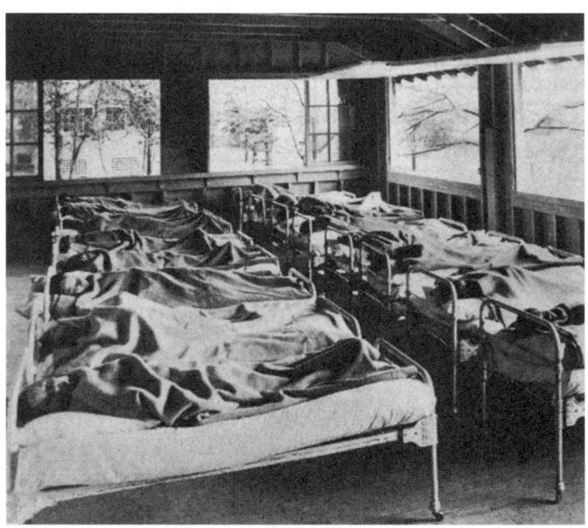

FIGURE 2.1 Open-air sleeping porch, southern exposure. Tuberculosis Preventorium for Children, Farmingdale, NJ. *Reprinted courtesy of J. Palmer Quimby, "The Tuberculosis Preventorium for Children, Farmingdale, N.J.," Modern Hospital 8: 177–179.*

members' vacation at the preventorium so that she never had to take a day off (Figure 2.1).[20]

While the child resided at the preventorium, nurses from the New York City health department or private nursing organizations such as the Henry Street Settlement conducted mandatory home visits and instructed parents on the importance of cleanliness and hygiene. When feasible, nurses facilitated sanatorium admission for the tubercular parent. Before a child's discharge, either Quimby or a public health nurse visited the home to make sure it met specified requirements. These might include recovery (and health practices and parenting behaviors deemed adequate) or death of the afflicted parent or be limited to a cleaner, more hygienic, better ventilated environment. Nurses followed up former patients indefinitely. As one Farmingdale report emphasized: "No child is returned from the Preventorium until the nurse reports home conditions safe. The children are *followed up* by a special Department of Health nurse for years. . . . Our purpose is to *permanently* save every child that comes to us."[21]

---

[20]Farmingdale Annual Report, 1927–1928, New York Historical Society; Farmingdale Annual Report, 1938, 1939, 1940, Howell Historical Society, Howell, New Jersey.

[21]Farmingdale Annual Report, 1912, Nathan Straus papers, box 8, Humanities and Social Sciences Library, Manuscripts and Archives Division, New York Public Library.

Despite the personal and professional isolation Quimby faced, her job provided a great deal of autonomy and satisfaction. Articulate and committed to her work, she published an article about Farmingdale in the journal *Modern Hospital*, an unusual accomplishment for a nurse of her era.[22] Local newspapers celebrated her efforts, a 1917 article in the New York *Evening Journal* illustrated Quimby's importance:

> Able physicians, generous philanthropists . . . help to make that admirable institution what it is. But let us not forget the mainspring of the watch. The mainstream of the preventorium [is] . . . Miss Quimby, general manager and boss of the institution, admirable type of woman who does things and keeps on doing them without losing patience, deserves the chief honors, in describing this home to which children come from the horror of consumption, to return in perfect health. . . . It is not gay work, receiving poor little half-starved children from the city. . . . It is not easy to be eternally patient, gentle, and affectionate with boys and girls that miss their mothers and cry themselves to sleep longing for the disease-infected home from which they have been rescued. . . . Miss Quinby [*sic*] is one of the noble women who do such work and enjoy doing it.[23]

The article did not mention one of Quimby's most important duties: helping to manage costs in order to keep the preventorium financially solvent. By 1926, she was busier than ever: The preventorium's average daily census that year was 166, more than double the capacity of its early days. Quimby supervised the institution's matron and growing number of employees, addressed issues related to the preventorium's operations as they arose, and determined which crises needed to be forwarded to Hess or the board of directors. She made sure that food and supplies got ordered, laundry got washed, and the physical plant remained in working order. Quimby also served as the link between parents and children, responding to inquiries from worried parents and making sure that children wrote home regularly.[24]

Eleven years before women won the right to vote, Quimby managed all aspects of a complex health care institution. In addition to the Farmingdale nurse's role as chief operating officer, educator, disciplinarian, counselor, and substitute mother, Quimby needed to attend carefully to children's health, monitoring their nutritional intake, weight, temperature, and other barometers

---

[22] J. Palmer Quimby, "The Tuberculosis Preventorium for Children, Farmingdale, N.J.," *Modern Hospital* 8 (March 1917): 177–179.

[23] Editorial, *New York Evening Journal*, June 14, 1917, box 16, Nathan Straus papers, box 16, Humanities and Social Sciences Library, Manuscripts and Archives Division, New York Public Library.

[24] Farmingdale Annual Report, 1927–1928, New York Historical Society.

of physical well-being. It was Quimby who decided when a child was ill enough for a physician to be notified, and it was she who decided which physician to contact. Her role grew especially powerful during the Great Depression in the 1930s. Preventorium staff received not only a salary, but free room and board, making it a highly attractive place to work. But it was Quimby who made hiring decisions and she who decided whether they stayed.

Children usually gained weight while institutionalized, and many returned home healthier. Nevertheless, preventoria operated under several flawed premises. The parent who was infected with TB was usually still in the home, often with other children. Health care providers knew that a bacterium caused TB, so it made little sense to leave others in the home to become infected. Also, the nurses and physicians involved hoped that the children's protracted stays away from their families could be used as an opportunity to indoctrinate the offspring of immigrants and the poor with middle-class American standards of hygiene and diet. Many nurses were not members of the upper or middle classes, yet they stood as links between these groups.

The therapeutic aim of building resistance to TB through a strict regimen of fresh air, ample nutrition, and education regarding health, morality, and good citizenship remained unchanged until the 1940s, even as scientific understanding of TB shifted and the idea of sending children away from their families declined in popularity. However, although the introduction of streptomycin in 1944, followed by isoniazid in 1952, meant that TB became a disease treatable with outpatient therapy, most institutions did not automatically close. Rather, they broadened admission criteria or attempted to cut expenses in order to remain in operation. At least one institution remained open until the 1970s.

CONCLUSION: UNDERSTANDING EVIDENCE IN "REAL TIME"

Why should nurses remember long-forgotten nursing interventions for a disease that afflicts few American children today? There are several reasons for doing so. First, the preventorium experiment and early twentieth-century TB public health nursing reveals an early instance not merely in which nurses and their work shaped health care policy and vice versa, but also of interdisciplinary collaboration between many different health care disciplines to address a major public health threat exemplified by the 1908 Tuberculosis Congress. Unfortunately, this practice dwindled during the twentieth century as each health care profession—including nursing—spent more and more time speaking to members of its own group. Today, a trend toward interdisciplinary collaboration is again being promoted for its cost-effectiveness and potential for societal benefit. As such, this case study reveals not only that meaningful cross-disciplinary collaboration is possible but also that there is also precedent for it.

The preventorium story is important to remember because the set of issues that led to the inception of the preventorium continue to pervade American society. The preventorium's founders and supporters struggled to translate new research into public health policy and clinical practice in an era of rapid social and scientific change. They debated how much intrusion should be allowed into family life and the boundaries between individual freedom and the need to protect the public's health. Preventorium founders also wrestled with concerns such as how best to help indigent families, what society "owes" children in terms of health and social welfare services, how much control parents should have over their own children, and who should decide what interventions are "in the best interest of the child." These topics remain as compelling at the start of the twenty-first century as they were at the beginning of the twentieth.[25]

Finally, the preventorium is also a cautionary tale worth remembering in the midst of the the childhood obesity epidemic. Many preventorium nurses (and physicians and public health officials) conflated practices supported by data that have endured, such as covering one's mouth when coughing or avoiding spitting, with other interventions that reflected ethnic or class-based prejudices such as disdain for certain foods or preset ideas concerning what constituted a healthy home. This reveals how difficult it is in "real time" to unpack evolving science from personal preference and even prejudice. This is particularly true for conditions, such as TB in 1909 and childhood obesity in 2009, with no simple cure, especially conditions for which self-control and "good" parenting have been put forward as important.

ACKNOWLEDGMENTS

An earlier version of this article was published in the Nursing History Review: C. A. Connolly, "Nurses: The Early Twentieth Century Tuberculosis Preventorium Movement's 'Connecting Link'." Nursing History Review 10 (2002): 127–157. The author is grateful to Springer Publishing Company for allowing parts of the 2002 article to be reproduced.

---

[25]Report of S. 1172, 108th Congress, Improved Nutrition and Physical Activity Act, http://thomas.loc.gov/cgi-bin/cpquery/T?&report=sr245&dbname=cp108 (accessed November 18, 2006).

CHAPTER 3

Treating Influenza 1918 and 2010: Recycled Interventions

Arlene W. Keeling

September 30, 2009

H1N1 FLU SURGE STARTS FULL THROTTLE . . . HOSPITALS UNDER SIEGE

> After months of warnings and frantic preparations, the second wave of the swine flu pandemic is starting to be felt around the country, as doctors, health clinics, hospitals and schools are reporting rapidly increasing numbers of patients experiencing flu symptoms. In Austin, so many parents are rushing their children to the Dell Children's Medical Center of Central Texas with swine flu symptoms that the hospital had to set up tents in the parking lot to cope with the onslaught. In Memphis, the Le Bonheur Children's Medical Center emergency room got so crowded with feverish, miserable youngsters that it had to do the same thing. . . .[1]

On September 30, 2009, the news about the spreading H1N1 influenza virus was grim. Medical centers in Texas and Tennessee were inundated with sick patients to the extent that hospital officials set up tents to house the overflow. The novel influenza virus was epidemic in Mexico and the United States and rapidly becoming pandemic. Public health personnel, physicians, and nursing personnel were concerned: The flu virus, in some cases mild but in

[1]*Pandemic Influenza News*, September 2009, http://emssolutionsinc.wordpress.com/2009/09 (accessed October 28, 2009).

other cases severe, could suddenly mutate to a more deadly form. Meanwhile, hospital officials faced a more pressing issue: They needed to increase the number of beds they had to care for those who were sickest. Setting up tents seemed to be the answer, one that was reminiscent of what hospital officials did almost a century earlier in Boston, Massachusetts, in August of 1918 when a deadly form of influenza hit that city. So was advising patients to stay home, rest, and drink fluids until the flu subsided; to cover coughs and sneezes, to wash hands, and to wear masks in public places. In fact, almost a century after the Great Flu of 1918, and despite major changes in medical and nursing therapeutics—including the availability of H1N1 vaccines and antiviral medications—much of the national and community response to the epidemic has been reminiscent of 1918.

This chapter examines the nursing and public health interventions used in the 1918 pandemic, noting how commonplace therapies (e.g., cough medicines, antipyretics, and fluids) and preventive measures (e.g., hand washing and the use of face masks), as well as social distancing activities (e.g., school closures and quarantine) and the expansion of hospital spaces, are among the flu interventions "recycled" for implementation today.[2] The hope is that this brief history will stimulate the reader's thinking about how so much has changed over the century and yet how much remains the same in the prevention and treatment of this highly infectious virus. It also notes the important role that the nursing profession had during this devastating pandemic.

THE 1918 FLU

The influenza pandemic of 1918 killed more than 40 million people worldwide and caused more than 675,000 deaths in the United States.[3] In 1918, the extremely high death rate—particularly among young adults—from a rare and highly contagious form of influenza was mysterious and frightening.

---

[2]Arlene Keeling and Mary Ramos, "The Role of Nursing History in Preparing Nursing for the Future," *Nursing and Health Care* 16, no. 1 (January/February 1995): 30–34.

[3]Fieser to Atkinson, January 15, 1941, re: Influenza Epidemic of 1918. National Archives and Record Administration—College Park (hereafter cited as NARA-CP) Records of the Red Cross. Epi Flu 803.11, box 557, 500.2—Influenza. (Jeffrey Taubenberger and co-workers at the U.S. Armed Forces Institute of Pathology showed that the 1918 flu was H1N1.) See also, Maurice R. Hilleman, "Realities and Enigmas of Human Viral Influenza: Pathogenesis, Epidemiology and Control," *Vaccine* 20 (2002): 3068–3087. According to Hilleman, Influenza A was discovered in 1933 (p. 3074) and the 1918 flu was H1N1. It killed more than 40 million people throughout the world.

Moreover, the nation was unprepared for the magnitude of the epidemic. Reflecting on the events of the fall of 1918, nurse leader Janet Geister later wrote: "We weren't ready in plans and resources, nor were we ready in our thinking. A country-wide epidemic was utterly inconceivable."[4] To complicate the situation, the United States had entered the war in Europe only a year earlier and thousands of physicians and nurses had been deployed overseas during the spring and summer of 1918. Only the few thousand public health and visiting nurses who had been spared deployment to the European front and classified as Home Defense Nurses were left to cope with the major epidemic that struck the United States that fall.

The 1918 flu (recently identified as H1N1) was called "Spanish flu" because Spain, neutral in the war, was one of the few countries to first admit it had a problem. Indeed, in the summer and fall of 1918, news of influenza in other parts of the world was difficult to access. In the interest of national security, the French, German, and British newspapers did not report the negative impact of flu on their troops. The Spanish press, on the other hand, did not hesitate to report the widespread impact of influenza among its citizens and hence the name.[5]

The virus was extremely contagious and sometimes deadly, particularly for pregnant women and young men between the ages of 20 and 40 years. The illness had an incubation of 1 to 2 days, a sudden onset followed by extreme prostration and fever, severe muscle pain, and bleeding from the nose and mouth. It was often accompanied by what physicians then labeled bronchopneumonia, in which case mortality was 60%–70%. Death sometimes occurred within 12 to 24 hours; at other times after a week or more.

In 1918, the primary treatment for flu was the provision of nursing care. Nurses sponged patients to reduce fever; provided them with soups and other liquid nourishment; covered them with warm, dry blankets; and opened windows to allow in fresh air. In severe cases, under medical orders, nurses sometimes administered oxygen or cardiac medications like digitalis. For the most part, however, nurses gave household remedies like aspirin and cough medicines, Listerine gargles, and mustard plasters.[6] They also provided nourishment, giving patients "gruels, cereals, milk toast, eggs, milk, etc." in small quantities.[7]

---

[4]Janet Geister, "The Flu Epidemic of 1918," *Nursing Outlook* 5, no. 10 (October 1957): 582–584. Geister was working with the Children's Bureau during the epidemic.

[5]Ibid., 171.

[6]Arlene Keeling, *Nursing and the Privilege of Prescription, 1893–2000* (Ohio: Ohio State University Press, 2007).

[7]"How to Care for Influenza and Pneumonia Patients," *The Public Health Nurse* 10, no. 7 (November 1918): 238–245 (quote, p. 244).

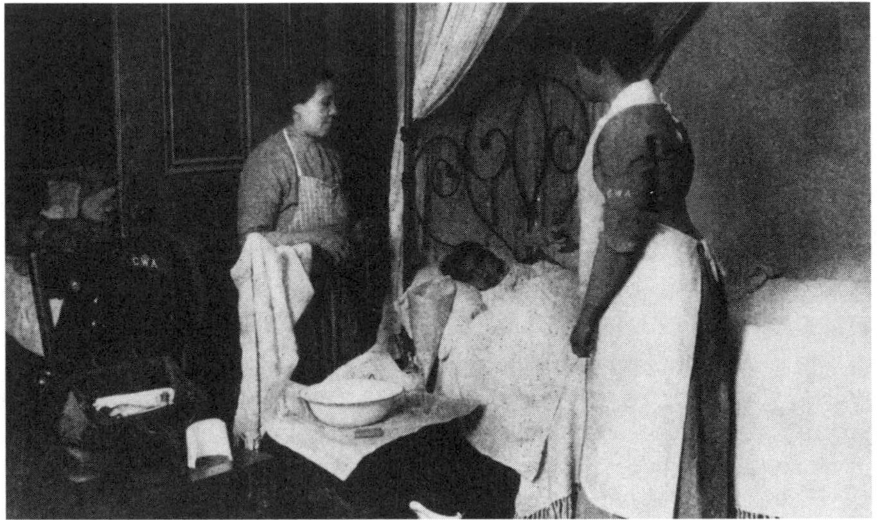

FIGURE 3.1 Child with flu. *Reprinted courtesy of the National Library of Medicine.*

In the United States, influenza first broke out in Kansas at a crowded military recruit camp and then spread rapidly as soldiers moved across the country. It erupted in Boston in late August and then in Philadelphia and New York in mid-September. By late September, city health officials were appealing to Washington, DC, for help, and on September 25, the American Red Cross National Committee met in the Capitol to implement the plan they had formulated a year earlier to address emergency situations within the U.S. borders. Afterward, Assistant Director of the Red Cross Nursing Division Clara Noyes telegraphed all Red Cross chapters: "Suggest you organize Home Defense nurses . . . to meet present epidemic. . . . Provide nurses with masks."[8]

Local Red Cross chapters responded immediately, forming committees to organize the nursing response, setting up volunteer motor corps and soup kitchens, and organizing women volunteers to make thousands of gauze masks. Public health nurses, school and industrial nurses, visiting nurse associations, and hospital nurses were essential to this plan; some had already been working for weeks to respond to the flu.

---

[8]Clara Noyes, "Memo to All Division Directors," September 24, 1918. NARA-CP, Epi Flu 803.11, box 689.

Within a matter of days, the epidemic spread south along the East Coast along transportation lines, striking Baltimore, Washington, Richmond, and smaller towns along the way. It then traveled west to Chicago and St. Louis, erupting in cities and small towns throughout the country and exploding in Seattle during the last week in September. By October 19, more than 4,000 new cases of flu were reported as far away as San Francisco.[9]

HOSPITAL OVERFLOW

Civilian hospitals were soon filled to capacity; 20-bed wards stretched to accommodate 40 to 50 patients. The experience of one student nurse who worked 12-hour shifts in a flu ward in New York was typical of what was occurring everywhere:

> . . . Almost overnight the hospital was inundated. . . . Wards were emptied hastily of patients convalescing from other ailments . . . only emergency operations were performed. Cots appeared down the center of wards . . . vacations all cancelled . . . classes disrupted. . . . Victims came on stretchers . . . their faces and nails as blue as huckleberries.[10]

In response, some cities and towns opened emergency hospitals in schools, warehouses, churches, or any available building.[11] According to one report from a public health nurse in South Dakota: ". . . for five weeks we used the dormitory and the State Normal School, then moved to an old residence. The patients were brought in from all over Lake County . . . many farm hands with pneumonia. We treated 175 cases with 4 deaths. . . ."[12]

In Brookline, a subdivision of Boston, officials set up an emergency open-air tent hospital.[13] Soon tent hospitals were commonplace as public health

---

[9]Alfred W. Crosby, *America's Forgotten Pandemic: The Influenza of 1918*, 2nd ed. (Cambridge: Cambridge University Press, 2003): 92–94.

[10]Dorothy Deming, "Influenza, 1918: Reliving the Great Epidemic," *American Journal of Nursing* 57, no. 10 (October 1957): 1308–1309.

[11]Southeastern Pennsylvania Chapter of the American Red Cross (ARC), *Report, September–October 1918*, NARA-CP, Epi Flu 803.11, box 689.

[12]"Some Side-Lights on the Influenza Epidemic," *Public Health Nurse* 1, no. 4 (April 1919): 300–304.

[13]J. Jackson, ARC Correspondence to Frank Person, ARC Washington, DC, October 4, 1918. NARA-CP, Epi Flu 803, box 688.

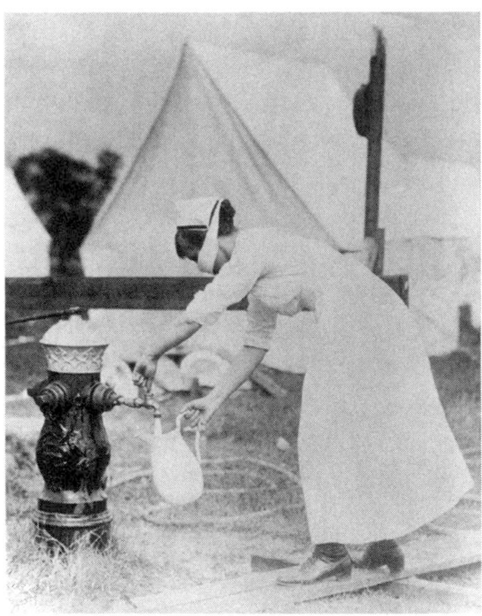

FIGURE 3.2 Nurse outside tent hospital, ca. 1918. *Reprinted courtesy of the National Archives.*

officials advocated "open-air" beds to prevent the spread of the highly contagious disease.

In most areas, despite the dire need for nurses and the widespread nature of the epidemic among all races, city and hospital officials maintained the commonly accepted social norm of racial segregation, separating African American patients into hospital wards (often in the basement) identified for them only. In other cases, separate buildings were used. For example, in Greenville, Mississippi, where more than 1,800 African Americans succumbed to the flu during the month of October, the local Red Cross chapter set up an emergency hospital for blacks only and put out a special call for black nurses.[14]

Soon all hospitals were reeling from the effects of the epidemic. The situation in Chicago was typical. On October 1, Cook County Hospital reported 260 influenza cases, 60 of which had arrived that day.[15] Provident Hospital, the hospital for the large black community on Chicago's South side, was also inundated.[16] In fact, the capacity of the hospitals was nearly exhausted and Chicago's

---

[14]"Help for the Colored People,"*The Weekly Democrat-Times*, October 22, 1918, 1.
[15]"All Flu Cases Quarantined by Order of City," *The Chicago Daily Tribune*, October 1, 1918.
[16]Vanessa Gamble, *Making a Place for Ourselves: The Black Hospital Movement, 1920–1945* (New York: Oxford University Press, 1995).

Commissioner of Health John Robertson ordered "every victim . . . to go to his home and stay there."[17] As was the case in cities and towns all over the country, most patients would have to be cared for at home.

PUBLIC HEALTH AND VISITING NURSING

With hospitals overflowing, public health nurses assumed the major responsibility for caring for the thousands who were ill. In cities, where immigrant ghettos were known to be "hives of sickness,"[18] nurses visited patients in their overcrowded tenement flats and row houses. In some cases, the nurses were the first and only ones to do so.[19] Director of the Henry Street Settlement Visiting Nurses Lillian Wald explained a situation in upper Harlem where the mother had flu, the father had lobar pneumonia, two children had measles, and one child was only 4 weeks old. The family, she said, "had been without care of any kind until the case was reported to the visiting nurse," adding, "this is a situation duplicated in hundreds of homes."[20]

In Chicago, The Visiting Nurse Association was also stretched thin, despite the fact that it had 93 nurses working out of 10 dispensaries scattered throughout the city.[21] As Assistant Superintendent Mary Westphal described: ". . . We were very hard hit on the west side of Chicago, and are still getting calls where entire families are ill. Dirty streets, dirty alleys and just as dirty houses . . . have made our work more than usually difficult."[22] Indeed, the nurses worked from early morning until late at night. By October 10, Chicago was reporting "1,421 cases of flu and 340 of pneumonia, with 72 deaths from pneumonia and 55 from influenza."

In rural areas, nurses called on families in distant farmhouses, log cabins, and shacks. There they did the best they could, often working in isolation to

---

[17]"Cases," *The Chicago Daily Tribune*, October 1, 1918.

[18]David Rosner, *Hives of Sickness: Public Health and Epidemics in New York City*. (New Brunswick, NJ: Rutgers University Press, 1995).

[19]Lavinia Dock, *Text-Book of Materia Medica for Nurses* (New York: G.P. Putnam's Sons, 1892), Preface.

[20]Lillian Wald, "Influenza: When the City Is a Great Field Hospital," *Survey* (February 14, 1920): 1 (reprint), LWC, NYPL, reel 2, box 3.

[21]"The Visiting Nurse Association (VNA) Substation Data," Chicago VNA Collection, Chicago History Museum, box 16, folders 1–3.

[22]Mary Westphal, "Society Women Work as Nurses in Flu Hospital,"*The Chicago Daily Tribune*, October 10, 1918.

care for entire poverty-stricken families. One African American nurse, Bessie B. Hawse, recounted her experience, noting:

> Eight miles from Talladega in the back woods, a colored [*sic*] family of ten were in bed and dying for the want of attention. No one would come near. I was asked by the health officer if I would go. I was glad of the opportunity. As I entered the little country cabin I found the mother dead in bed. Three children buried the week before. The father and remainder of the family running a temperature of 102–104. Some had influenza, others had pneumonia. . . . I rolled up my sleeves and killed chickens and began to cook. I forgot I was not a cook, but I only thought of saving lives. I milked the cow, gave medicine, and did everything I could to help. . . .[23]

NURSING TREATMENTS

In all settings, nurses provided the most basic care. They bathed patients and dressed them in flannel pneumonia jackets, changed linens, and checked temperatures, pulse, and respirations. They also gave patients fluids and fed them broth, eggnogs, and milk. Following medical orders, or relying on their own nursing expertise and making do with what they had on hand, the nurses administered such treatments as ice packs and aspirin to reduce fever and mustard plasters and cough syrups to alleviate lung congestion.[24] In hospitals, treatment was a bit more sophisticated. According to one nurse: ". . . we gave heart and respiratory stimulants, but we were forever balancing the advantages of forcing fluids against the disadvantages of edema, as kidneys or heart became overtaxed and the lungs showed congestion. . . ."[25]

"CONTAGIOUS NURSING" AND MASKS

Key to the nurses' routine was the use of gauze masks mandated by the Red Cross, to be worn "constantly in congested homes, [when] . . . doing anything

---

[23]Darlene C. Hine, *Black Women in the Nursing Profession: A Documentary History.* (New York: Garland Publishing, 1985).
[24]What the Boston Metropolitan Chapter of the Red Cross accomplished during the epidemic (November 18, 1918): 2–3. NARA-CP, Epi Flu 803.11, box 689, Massachusetts. See also, Arlene Keeling, "Chapter 1: Midway between the Pharmacist and the Physician," in *Nursing and the Privilege of Prescription, 1893–2000* (Ohio: Ohio State University Press, 2007), 1–27.
[25]Deming, "Influenza, 1918," 1308–1309.

for the patient."[26] It was a mandate created in the hope of preventing the nurses and others from contracting the fatal disease. Unfortunately, it was of minimal usefulness, and in fact, resulted in a set of tedious procedures to be completed by the nurses. As Superintendent Edna Foley later recorded:

> We began by using a stitched mask with four strings. This involved carrying two bags, one for fresh and one for soiled masks, and a supply of about sixteen masks for each nurse. It also required someone to boil these masks and dry them daily, and before long we conceived the idea of folding squares of gauze on the bias, making strips of six thicknesses of gauze, which were tied over the face or pinned to the hair. Each one of these improvised masks was folded in a paper towel, and after the mask was discarded, it was burned.[27]

Indeed the use of masks and isolation procedures learned in nursing school was widespread during the epidemic. Working as superintendent of an emergency hospital set up in the State Normal School in the small town of Madison, South Dakota, nurse Merlin Wilkins implemented "strict contagious nursing . . . learned in Chicago," in which the nurses "wore caps, gowns, and masks all the time while in patients' rooms."[28]

HEALTH EDUCATION

Part of the nurses' role included health education. All over the country, nurses taught families basic hygienic practices, educating them about the importance of getting proper nutrition, avoiding crowds, covering coughs and spitting into handkerchiefs, boiling soiled linens, and opening windows for fresh air. They also taught basic principles of nursing the sick and instructing people about the signs and symptoms of flu, its treatment, and how it spread. To reach patients and their families in remote rural farms and villages, Jane A. Delano, Director of Nursing for the American Red Cross, wrote a series of articles based on her nursing experience, outlining "details of practical help" in caring for flu victims. These were published in

---

[26]"How to Care for Influenza and Pneumonia Patients," *Public Health Nursing* 10, no. 7 (November 1918): 238–245.

[27]Edna Foley, "Department of Public Health Nursing, Illinois," *American Journal of Nursing* 19, no. 3 (December 1918): 189–200 (quote, p. 192).

[28]"Some Side-Lights," 304.

newspapers that "circulated through the rural districts and isolated Western communities."[29]

In an attempt to stop the spread of the disease, city health officials mandated the use of masks in public places, and nurses taught families how to use them.

ISOLATION AND QUARANTINES

Across the country, health officials instituted quarantine and isolation of sick patients to prevent the spread of disease. On September 26, Richmond's (Virginia) Chief Health Officer Roy K. Flannagan met with other health directors to establish quarantine guidelines for schoolchildren affected by influenza. According to those guidelines, children were to be kept away from school "until the attending physician has found that all danger has passed."[30] And, on the morning of October 6, 1918, the residents of the small central Virginia city of Lynchburg awoke to an alarming newspaper headline restricting children to their homes and closing schools, churches, and moving-picture shows. According to the proclamation issued by Lynchburg's mayor:

> I have been informed this afternoon that Spanish Influenza is increasing rapidly in this city. In view of that fact, it is earnestly hoped that all residents of this community will co-operate with the health authorities and physicians in doing what they can to check the spreading of the disease. Parents are urged to keep their children on their own premises. All visiting by either children or adults should be eliminated. It is believed that if the people generally will remain at home as far as practicable, the spreading of the disease will be more easily checked. The orders of the board of health with reference to the closing of the schools, churches, theatres, moving picture shows and public meetings of all kinds will be strictly enforced by the police until further orders from the board.[31]

Much the same was the case in other small towns and large cities. In Topeka, Kansas (population 60,000) the Board of Health issued closing orders on its "schools, business establishments, churches, and places of amusement."[32] When the flu struck San Francisco in mid-October, several weeks

---

[29]Katherine Wood, "Battling with 'Flu'," *The Red Cross Magazine* (1919): 11–17 (quote, p. 16).
[30]"Some Side-Lights," 304.
[31]"Board of Health Issues Drastic Closing Orders," *The News*, October 6, 1918.
[32]"Some Side-Lights," 301.

after it was widespread on the East Coast, the State Board of Health ordered all moving-picture houses and other theaters throughout the state closed as a precautionary measure. The board stopped short of closing schools "wherever the teachers could be relied upon to immediately exclude any child appearing with symptoms."[33] Their rationale: It was safer to have children in school than roaming the streets.

CONCLUSION

While almost a century has passed since the devastating 1918 influenza pandemic struck the United States, many of the medical and nursing interventions for the prevention of its spread and the treatment of the disease remain the same. In 1918, public health officials, physicians, and nurses recommended isolation of patients, hand washing, covering coughs, and using masks to prevent its spread. They also advocated health-promoting behaviors like fresh air and exercise and nutritious diets as preventive measures. When patients did succumb to the illness, treatments were simple and included warm liquids, aspirin, cough syrups, and gargles. When hospitals were inundated with victims, outdoor tents were set up to expand bed capacity.

Today, despite the availability of antiviral medications, flu vaccines, and high-tech interventions for respiratory distress, much of the population suffering from flu turns to the simple remedies used in the past: aspirin and its modern counterparts Tylenol and Advil; cough medicine and gargles; hand washing; and the use of masks. They also look to nurses, public health officials, and physicians for published guidelines on how to safeguard against the flu and what to do should they catch it.[34] In many towns and cities, schools are closed to prevent its spread. However, when the virus spreads despite the best precautionary measures and thousands of people succumb, tents are set up to expand hospitals' capacity. Indeed, "recycled" solutions from the past may prove to be useful interventions during twenty-first-century epidemics.

---

[33]"State Health Board Closes All Theaters," *San Francisco Chronicle*, October 19, 1918, 6.

[34]United States Public Health Service, *Supplement No. 34 to Public Health Reports: "Spanish Influenza"* (September 28, 1918).

CHAPTER 4

"An Obstinate and Sometimes Gangrenous Sore": Prevention and Nursing Care of Bedsores, 1900 to the 1940s

Helen Zuelzer

On a spring day in 1995, after a fall while horseback riding, actor Christopher Reeve, star of the movie *Superman,* was paralyzed from the neck down because of a severe cervical spinal cord injury.[1]

Prior to his accident, Mr. Reeve was athletic and in excellent physical shape. After the accident, he was unable to move or breathe on his own. Mr. Reeve, however, could afford the best medical care and state-of-the-art rehabilitation, including 24-hour-a-day nursing care. When interviewed on a television program in 2002 about the remarkable progress he had made in the years since his accident, he acknowledged his ability to pay for this kind of care. "I'm privileged," he stated. "I have a staff. I have the equipment. . . ." He also talked of his experience with pressure ulcers. ". . . I've had my share of pressure sores," he admitted. ". . . I have had some really bad ones. . . ."[2]

---

[1]Douglas Marten, "Christopher Reeve, 52, Symbol of Courage, Dies," *New York Times*, (October 12, 2004), http://query.nytimes.com/gst/fullpage.html?res=9504E0DA113BF931A25753C1A9629C8B63&ref=christopher_reeve (accessed March 25, 2010) (hereafter cited as Marten, "Christopher Reeve," *New York Times*).

[2]Larry King Live, "Christopher and Dana Reeve Interview from Larry King" (September 24, 2002), http://sci.rutgers.edu/forum/showthread.php?t=16567 (accessed March 25, 2010).

Despite his access to excellent care, Christopher Reeve died from an infected pressure ulcer on October 12, 2004, at the age of 52.[3]

A 1926 definition of bedsore as ". . . an obstinate and sometimes gangrenous sore, caused by pressure. . .,"[4] remains appropriate today. Pressure injury of tissues; the extent to which such injury is preventable; and the relationships among injury, preventive measures, and their relationship to nursing care have remained problematic for over a century. While pressure ulcers have long been recognized as a significant source of suffering and even death, they have, of late, taken on new significance due to recent federal legislation based on the premise that pressure ulcers are preventable.[5] Since October 2008, the Center for Medicare and Medicaid Services no longer pays acute care facilities for the care, treatment, or extra days of hospitalization related to severe pressure ulcers that occur as a result of, or during, that hospitalization.

Pressure ulcers, once called bedsores, remain an enigma and a scourge to the individuals who develop them and to nurses and others who seek to prevent their occurrence. Thus, this "obstinate . . . sore"[6] has not only not gone away; the implications of its occurrence have increased exponentially. This chapter explores the role of nursing in the prevention and treatment of pressure ulcers during the first half of the twentieth century. It seeks to explicate the knowledge and role of nurses in maintaining skin integrity, in identifying risk factors, and in using nursing interventions and therapeutic modalities, increasingly informed by scientific and technologic advances.

---

[3]Marten, "Christopher Reeve," *New York Times*.

[4]W. A. Newman Dorland, ed. *American Pocket Medical Dictionary*, 13th ed. (Philadelphia, WB Saunders, 1926), quote p. 95 (hereafter cited as Dorland, *American Medical Dictionary*), "bedsore—an obstinate and sometimes gangrenous sore, caused by pressure of the body of a patient against the bed."

[5]U.S. Department of Health and Human Services, Centers for Medicare and Medicaid Services 42 CFR Parts 411, 412, 413, and 489 Medicare Program, " Changes to the Hospital Inpatient Prospective Payment Systems and Fiscal Year 2008 Rates; Final Rule," *Federal Register*, Part II, 72, no. 162 (2007): 47200–47218. http://www.regulations.gov/search/Regs/home.html#docketDetail?R=CMS-2007-0148. Effective October 2008 (accessed November 20, 2007). According to Center for Medicare and Medicaid Services, reimbursement changes, the considerable costs of extended hospitalization, treatment modalities, and treatment of pressure ulcer–related complications associated with post-hospital admission pressure ulcers will be borne by the hospitals themselves. Medicare dollars will no longer be spent for the care associated with postadmission pressure ulcers. As part of the Deficit Reduction Act of 2005, the Secretary of Health and Human Services was mandated to select hospital-acquired secondary diagnoses or complications, which would no longer be reimbursed by Medicare. Conditions selected for this "no reimbursement list" met criteria that included high cost/high burden, as well as reasonably preventable via utilization of identified evidence-based guidelines.

[6]Dorland, *American Medical Dictionary*, quote p. 95.

BEDSORES AND NURSING ACCOUNTABILITY

Nurses and others have long debated the avoidability of bedsores and nurses' accountability should they occur. Isabel Hampton, superintendent of nurses at Johns Hopkins Hospital and a founder of the National League of Nursing Education,[7] explicitly wrote about this in *Nursing: Its Principles and Practice. For Hospital and Private Use*, one of the earliest textbooks of nursing, published in 1903. "To guard against bed-sores is one of the first injunctions given to a nurse who is entrusted with the care of a bed patient," she explained. "It is just here that good or bad nursing tells, and the development of a bed-sore while the patient is under a nurse's care gives ground for severe criticism."[8]

Numerous nursing texts reflected the theme of poor nursing care as the root cause of bedsores, with the nurse culpable due to her neglect or lack of effort. Anna Maxwell, superintendent of Presbyterian Hospital School of Nursing and former superintendent of the Boston Training School for Nurses, and her coauthor Amy Pope, a nurse educator, formerly at the Presbyterian Hospital, very explicitly stated in their 1914 nursing text *Practical Nursing: A Textbook for Nurses* that "except in very rare instances, the nurses in charge of a patient are responsible if she [the patient] develops a bed-sore."[9] Virna Young, a nurse educator, and Pope were even more emphatic in their 1935 nursing textbook. Should a patient develop a bedsore, they wrote, the nurse was responsible, ". . . and should feel thoroughly disgraced. . . ."[10]

Other nurse educators espoused similar views. For example, Georgiana Sanders, a former matron in England and former superintendent of nurses at the Polyclinic Hospital in Philadelphia and Massachusetts General Hospital, admonished nursing students in *Modern Methods in Nursing*, written in 1918,

---

[7]Martin Kaufman, ed. Joellen Watson Hawkins, Loretta P. Higgins, and Alice Howell Friedman, contrib. eds. *Dictionary of American Nursing Biography* (New York: Greenwood Press, 1988), 312–313. Isabel Hampton Robb, as the first superintendent of the Johns Hopkins School of Nursing was instrumental in shaping nursing education through a standardized rigorous curriculum.

[8]Isabel Adams Hampton, *Nursing: Its Principles and Practice. For Hospital and Private Use* (Cleveland, OH: E.C. Koeckert, 1903), 118–130, quote p. 126 (hereafter cited as Hampton, *Nursing Principles and Practice*).

[9]Anna Caroline Maxwell and Amy Elizabeth Pope, *Practical Nursing: A Text-Book for Nurses* (New York: G.P. Putnam's Sons, 1914), quote p. 172.

[10]Amy E. Pope and Virna M. Young, *The Art and Principles of Nursing* (New York: G.P. Putnam's Sons, 1935), quote p. 70 (hereafter cited as Pope and Young, *Art and Principles of Nursing*). These authors use the term "pressure sores," whereas earlier texts utilized the term "bedsore."

". . . it cannot be too emphatically laid before the pupil that for a patient in her charge to acquire a bed-sore points to culpable neglect on her part, so rare are the cases in which it may be considered unpreventable."[11] Irene Kelley, a nurse educator and director of several schools of nursing in the Midwest, reiterated these sentiments in the 1926, 1936, and 1942 editions of her book *Textbook of Nursing Technique*.[12]

Other authors unequivocally posited nurses' accountability for bedsores. For example, in two editions of her text *Text Book of the Principles and Practice of Nursing*, written in 1922 and 1937, Bertha Harmer, Director of the School for Graduate Nurses, McGill University and former assistant professor at Yale University School of Nursing, wrote that "the prevention of bedsores is entirely the responsibility of the nurse. . . . Bedsores are rarely unpreventable and are usually due to carelessness."[13] In the 1939 edition of the text, she added that development of a pressure sore reflected poorly on nursing care.[14] Ella Rothweiler, a nurse educator, and physician colleagues John Coulter and Felix Jansey added to this chorus in their editions of the nursing text titled *The Science and Art of Nursing*, changed to *The Art and Science of Nursing*, in 1940, admonishing students that, "To permit a patient to develop a bedsore is, in most instances, a disgrace to the nurse in charge as well as to the nursing staff."[15]

Yet other authors acknowledged that the relationship between nursing accountability and blame should a bedsore occur was not always straightforward. For example, Charlotte Brown, a nurse educator at Boston City Hospital, blamed bedsores on poor nursing care, but at the same time, she noted that they may not have been preventable. "There is nothing which tends to show poor nursing care than does a bed-sore, for they may in the majority of cases

---

[11]Georgiana J. Sanders, *Modern Methods in Nursing* (Philadelphia, PA: W.B. Saunders Company, 1918), 76–82, quote p. 77 (hereafter cited as Sanders, *Modern Methods*).

[12]Irene Kelley, *Text-book of Nursing Technique* (Philadelphia, PA: W.B. Saunders, 1926), 42–43 (hereafter cited as Kelley, *Text-book of Nursing*). These sentiments were later reiterated by Irene Kelley in the1936 (p. 44) and 1942 (p. 87) editions of the text: "The prevention of pressure sores is one of the most important duties of a nurse. With the right kind of nursing care a patient will rarely develop them. Except in unusual cases a nurse should feel that she is responsible for the condition and that she has not put forth the effort necessary to prevent them."

[13]Bertha Harmer, *Textbook of the Principles and Practice of Nursing* (New York: The MacMillan Company, 1922), quote p. 64 (hereafter cited as Harmer, *Textbook of the Principles*); 1928: quote p. 77; 1934: quote p. 98; 1939: quote p. 368.

[14]Ibid., 1939: p. 368.

[15]Jean White, ed. *The Science and Art of Nursing* by Ella Rothweiler with contributions by John Coulter and Felix Jansey (Philadelphia, PA: F.A. Davis, 1935), quote p. 213. Ibid., 1937: quote p. 213. Quote in later version in Ella Rothweiler and Jean White, *The Art and Science of Nursing* (Philadelphia: F.A. Davis, 1940), quote p. 183.

be avoided," she noted in 1914 in the text *The Junior Nurse.*[16] Yet, earlier she acknowledged "bed-sores, in many instances, may be prevented, while in some cases they cannot, in spite of all care."[17] Later, Ralph Colp, instructor of surgery at Columbia University, and Manelva Keller, former chief operating room nurse and anesthetist at St. Luke's Hospital in New York, wrote in their 1929 text *Textbook of Surgical Nursing* that bedsores were ". . . always a sad commentary on nursing care even though at times they are absolutely unavoidable."[18]

Some authors indicated that bedsores were not always preventable. Hampton in 1903, in the text *Nursing: Its Principles and Practice*, described that bedsores "resulting from malnutrition of the entire system (which) . . . even with the utmost care . . . are sometimes unavoidable."[19] Surgeons Willard Bartlett and C. R. Fancher noted in their book *The After Treatment of Surgical Patients* that bedsores were not always preventable in paralyzed patients.[20] Later, when discussing nursing care of the patient with paralysis in their 1935 nursing text *Surgical Nursing*, Hugh Cabot, a physician affiliated with the Mayo Clinic and Mary Giles, Associate Professor of Nursing Education at Vanderbilt University, also suggested that, ". . . it is not possible to avoid the development of pressure sores . . . since the vitality of the skin is abnormally diminished as the result of the paralysis . . . in spite of the most skillful and painstaking care."[21]

PREVENTION OF BEDSORES

Identification of Risk Factors

Early-twentieth-century nurses knew of the risk factors associated with the development of bedsores. As Harriett Higbee wrote in a 1901 article in the *American Journal of Nursing*, patients were at risk "if the skin is inactive, as

---

16Charlotte A. Brown, *The Junior Nurse* (Philadelphia, PA: Lea & Febiger, 1914), quote p. 95 (hereafter cited as Brown, *Junior Nurse*).
17Ibid., quote p. 93.
18Ralph Colp and Manelva Keller, *Textbook of Surgical Nursing, New Second Edition* (New York: The Macmillan Company, 1929), quote p. 188.
19Hampton, *Nursing Principles and Practice*, quote p. 126.
20Willard Bartlett and C. R. Fancher, "Postoperative Treatment in Old Age," in *The After Treatment of Surgical Patients*, ed. Willard Bartlett and Collaborators, 647–653, 652 (St. Louis, MO: C.V. Mosby Co, 1920) (hereafter cited as Bartlett and Fancher, *After Treatment of Surgical Patients*).
21Hugh Cabot and Mary Giles, *Surgical Nursing* (Philadelphia, PA: W.B. Saunders, 1935), quote pp. 223–224 (hereafter cited as Cabot and Giles, *Surgical Nursing*).

in paralysis, or there is frequent or constant moisture from perspiration or involuntary evacuations of urine or feces, the alcohol and boric acid, etc., are of very little value. . . ."[22] In 1903, Hampton recognized that risk for bedsores differed from patient to patient and noted that ". . . the danger of such an occurrence varies with the nature of the disease and the weight of the patient."[23] Extremes in body size, both thin and obese, were increasingly recognized as predisposing to bedsores. Nurse educators, Pope and Young, writing in 1935, also commented that obesity, ". . . favors the development of pressure sores by increasing the weight of the body upon the mattress and, as extreme fatness is sometimes the result of faulty metabolism, the tissues of an obese person may be poorly nourished."[24] Bedpans also compromised skin integrity. In 1916, Elizabeth Smart implicated the enamel bedpan as damaging to tissues, and compromising ". . . a bed-sore that was endeavoring to heal."[25] New technology in the form of new bedpan designs, such as the "Perfection" pan and the rubber slipper, were hailed as advances as they were easier on the patient's skin.[26]

Elderly and paralyzed patients confined to bed were known to be at risk for a bedsore.[27] Eleanor Barton, nurse author of a text on caring for the chronically ill, noted that paralyzed patients

> . . . have a special tendency to bed-sores, owing first, to their general state of malnutrition; secondly, to the pressure on the different parts owing to the helplessness of the patient; thirdly, to the constant irritation to the skin caused by incontinence. . . .[28]

Nurses also knew of areas on the body at risk for bedsores. In her *Textbook of Nursing Technique*, nurse educator Irene Kelley identified areas at risk for bedsores as ". . . bony prominences . . . back of the head and ears in infants . . . between the folds of the abdomen under the breasts and on the buttocks in obese patients." She also identified susceptible individuals as ". . . emaciated

---

[22]Harriet Higbee, "Practical Points on Private Nursing: Backs and Mouths," *American Journal of Nursing* 1, no. 5 (May 1901): 336–338; quote p. 336 (hereafter cited as Higbee, "Practical Points").
[23]Hampton, *Nursing Principles and Practice*, 118–130, quote p. 126.
[24]Pope and Young, *Art and Principles of Nursing*, 68–71, quote p. 68.
[25]Catherine Smart, *Bed-sores: Their Prevention and Cure* (London, UK: Jon Bale Sons & Danielsson, 1916), 29–36, quote p. 29 (hereafter cited as Smart, *Bed-sores*).
[26]Ibid., 29–36.
[27]Bartlett and Fancher, *After Treatment of Surgical Patients*, pp. 647–653.
[28]Eleanor Barton, *The Nursing of Chronic Patients* (London, UK: The Scientific Press, 1920), quote pp. 86–87 (hereafter cited as Barton, *Chronic Patients*).

and obese patients. . . . Those whose vitality is low . . . who have involuntary micturition and defecation . . . whose condition is such that the circulation is impaired, due to certain kinds of heart disease and paralysis." She also named those "suffering from faulty metabolism."[29]

Preventative Treatments

Cleansing of the skin, often in conjunction with massage, was both a key preventive strategy and an early treatment employed at the first sign of a bedsore. Skin-cleansing regimes, as described in 1901 by Higbee, were especially important when the patient had urinary or fecal incontinence:

> . . . the back should be washed with soap and water every six or eight hours, or after every involuntary evacuation, and thoroughly rubbed with a small amount of some oily substance as castor oil, camphorated oil, or a mixture like the following: (Mutton tallow, olive oil and carbolic acid). If the skin needs a great deal of stimulation, camphorated oil or better still castor oil. . . .[30]

Hampton also advocated preventive measures. She believed such an approach "consists in absolute cleanliness and the removal of pressure. The back and shoulders should be bathed night and morning, and gentle friction employed to keep the skin clean and active. . . ."[31] The importance of skin cleansing as a means of preventing bedsores was also echoed in the nursing text *A Quiz Book of Nursing: For Teachers and Students* written by Amy Pope and coauthor Thirza Pope, a former supervisor of the Visiting Nurses of New York, published in 1919:

> If possible, the whole body should be bathed every day, if this is not possible, it should be done twice a week at least. . . . Those parts where bedsores are likely to form, as the lower part of the spine, the shoulders, heels, and elbows, should be washed twice a day with warm water and soap and rubbed with alcohol and massaged. If bedsores seem imminent, this treatment must be repeated every four hours.[32]

In an attempt to actively prevent bedsores, various products were applied to the skin. Rubbing the skin with alcohol was a cornerstone of bedsore

---

[29]Kelley, *Text-book of Nursing*, 1926: quote p. 42; 1936: quote p. 44; 1942: quote p. 87.
[30]Higbee, "Practical Points," 336–338; quote p. 336.
[31]Hampton, *Nursing Principles and Practice*, 118–130, quote p. 127.
[32]Amy E. Pope and Thirza A. Pope, *A Quiz Book of Nursing for Teachers and Students* (New York: G.P. Putnam's Sons, 1919), 9–10, quote p. 9.

prevention. According to one materia medica text, "locally applied, alcohol is mildly irritating and cooling to the skin. . . . Such solutions harden and toughen the skin where exposed to pressure or mechanical irritation, and . . . prevent bedsores."[33] Hampton, in 1903 recommended the use of alcohol in caring for the skin:

> The back and shoulders should be bathed night and morning . . . afterwards rubbed with a 50 per cent solution of alcohol to harden the skin; and finally the parts are dusted thoroughly with some kind of powder which will absorb the moisture . . . the oxide-of-zinc powder or bismuth mixed with borax are of equal value.[34]

Still other preventive regimes were promoted. Surgeon George Crary and colleagues, in the text *In Sickness and in Health: A Manual of Domestic Medicine and Surgery, Hygiene, Dietetics, and Nursing*, written in 1916, recommended cleansing of the skin with soap and water followed by the application of alcohol and a particularly prepared powder to toughen the skin. This powder of

> . . . equal parts of oxide of zinc and starch or talcum powder is useful when applied sparingly. . . . A preparation of equal parts of collodion and castor oil painted over the surface forms an artificial skin and sometimes prevents a breaking down of the tissues.[35]

In 1920, Eleanor Barton, writing about the care of chronically ill patients, offered still more ointments that, together with skin cleansing, would prevent bedsores.

> . . . at least four-hourly . . . back and pressure points (are) . . . well washed . . . dried, and then rubbed or massaged . . . using a circulatory movement; this relieves the stagnant condition of the skin and promotes better circulation . . . rub in ointment—either zinc, or zinc and castor oil, or zinc and benzoin—. . . to form . . . a temporary mackintosh over the skin.[36]

---

[33]A. L. Muirhead and Edith P. Brodie, *Materia Medica for Nurses* (St. Louis, MO: C.V. Mosby, 1924), quote pp. 94–95.

[34]Hampton, *Nursing Principles and Practice,* quote p. 127.

[35]George W. Crary, et al. *In Sickness and in Health, A Manual of Domestic Medicine and Surgery,Hygiene Dietetics, and Nursing: Dealing in a Practical Way with the Problems Relating to the Maintenance of Health, The Prevention and Treatment of Disease, and the Most Effective Aid in Emergencies* (New York: D. Appleton and Company, 1912), quote p. 917 (hereafter cited as Crary et al., *In Sickness and in Health).*

[36]Barton, *Chronic Patients, quote* pp. 83–84.

Cleansing and toughening of the skin was also advocated by Cabot and Giles in caring for paralyzed patients, in 1935.[37] Harmer, in 1937, also advocated rubbing with alcohol to stimulate replacement of stagnant venous blood with arterial blood "frequently . . . three times a day . . . or every hour as the case demands."[38] However, in 1942, a new method for the prevention of bedsores was reported. This new "Paste" method, in which calamine was patted on the tissues and allowed to dry, was said to be more effective than previously used modalities that had come to include mutton tallow and infrared lamps.[39]

Pressure, Crumbs, and Wrinkles

While pressure was cited as a main factor in causing bedsores, crumbs and wrinkles in the sheets, coupled with moisture and irritation, were also believed to be important. Nursing measures mitigated these factors. For example, Hampton recommended the use of a rubber or cotton ring, and turning the patient, as well as keeping sheets, ". . . perfectly smooth and dry under the patient: sometimes even a slight wrinkle will produce redness and tenderness."[40] Crary identified several risk factors for skin injury and possible solutions:

> . . . the back should receive attention from the very beginning of the illness. Moisture, wrinkles, and crumbs are the commonest enemies to be combated. Moisture softens the skin; wrinkles and crumbs irritate and roughen it. . . . Frequent changes of linen, pads made from oakum or jute placed in old muslin or cheese cloth, or large sheets of Japanese paper. . . .[41]

Eleanor Barton, in 1920, espoused a more comprehensive approach that included turning and pressure relief. She addressed the "anxieties," that is, the "three b's—bowels, bladder, back" of caring for paralyzed patients. She wrote:

> As to irritation, the chief causes are . . . incontinence, rucks in the mackintosh, crumbs in the bed, or if the draw-sheet or end of the nightdress is allowed to remain in folds directly under the points of pressure. . . .[42]

---

[37]Cabot and Giles, *Surgical Nursing*, 223.
[38]Harmer, *Textbook of the Principles*, quote p. 101.
[39]Mary Weston, "The Paste Treatment of Bed Sores," *American Journal of Nursing* 40, no. 4 (1940): 388–390 (hereafter cited as Weston, "Paste Treatment").
[40]Hampton, *Nursing Principles and Practice*, quote p. 127.
[41]Crary et al., *In Sickness and in Health*, quote p. 916 and p. 917.
[42]Barton, *Chronic Patients*, quote pp. 83–84.

Technologies for Pressure Relief

Turning and repositioning patients at varying intervals were paramount in bedsore prevention. Nurses showed great ingenuity in utilizing available materials for the purpose of pressure redistribution. Higbee discussed early measures for relieving pressure at length:

> . . . the relief of pressure by the use of air-cushions, cotton-pads, pillows, water-bed and frequent change of position where that is possible . . . a simple, inexpensive contrivance used to relieve pressure of heel, elbow, and ear. It is a pig's bladder, filled two-thirds full of either warm or cold water . . . tied securely and placed under a cotton ring.[43]

Hampton continued to advocate pressure relief by means of rubber or cotton rings and changing position.[44] While Crary and colleagues promulgated changing position as the most important measure for relieving pressure, and identified several other pressure-relieving modalities such as:

> Air pillows, folded sheets, pillows made of hair, rubber rings covered with bandages to prevent moisture on the surface, rings made of batting or sheet wadding wound with bandages . . . rings can be made to fit any part of the body, from a tiny one small enough to prevent pressure upon the ear to one large enough to support the buttock . . . (it) often prevents the much-dreaded bedsore.[45]

Other technologies were also available. One 1916 device, the "Skeffington's Patent Recumbent Invalid Lifter," provided another means of relieving pressure. This contrivance, promoted as solving both the bedsore and bedpan problem, suspended the patient above the bed in a lying position by means of ropes and pulleys. Water and air mattresses were also offered as measures available for pressure relief.[46] Nurse Georgiana Sanders, in a 1918 nursing text, recommended the use of rubber rings inflated with air "just sufficiently," and ". . . small rings of many sizes may be cut out of muslin and stuffed with tow. . . ." She also advocated the use of an air-bed or water bed for emaciated patients.[47]

---

[43]Higbee, "Practical Points," 336–338; quote p. 336.
[44]Hampton, *Nursing Principles and Practice*, 118–129.
[45]Crary et al., *In Sickness and in Health*, quote p. 916 and p. 917.
[46]Smart, *Bed-sores*, 47–52.
[47]Sanders, *Modern Methods*, quote pp. 81–82.

TREATMENT OF BEDSORES

During the early twentieth century, various topical agents were the mainstay of bedsore treatment. Use of topical modalities was increasingly guided by a growing knowledge of wound care to promote wound healing. As early as 1901, wounds were filled with lightly fluffed and moist dressings, eliminating dead space and promoting moist wound healing.[48] Later, judicious use of cytotoxic agents, damaging to healthy tissues, was advocated and the use of moist wound-healing principles were evident. Emerging scientific knowledge included wound care based on wound assessment and characteristics of the wound, with bedsores characterized as chronic "stalled" wounds. The removal of necrotic tissue by means of chemical, mechanical, and sharp debridement was recognized as promoting healing. And surgical interventions, including skin grafts, became available as a means of wound closure.

The volume and variety of wound care remedies utilized exemplify the strong desire and effort expended to be rid of these "obstinate. . . sores."[49] For example, Higbee advised that the bedsore be:

> . . . cleansed . . . with boric-acid solution, normal salt solution, or sterile water; then gently painted with oxide of zinc ointment made into liquid form by the addition of olive oil, castor-oil, and balsam of Peru in equal parts, or castor oil alone[e]. . . . If there is necrotic tissue or suppuration present . . . irrigate the cavity once daily with peroxide of hydrogen—one glass syringeful—followed by normal salt solution, boric-acid solution, or sterile water . . . apply a hot boric-acid dressing—one inch thick—every four hours until the wound is clean. If the stimulation of the tissues is needed, fill the cavity with a sterile dressing saturated with balsam of Peru and castor oil in equal parts, bovinine, castor oil, or camphorated oil. . . .[50]

Hampton offered additional remedies tailored to the tissue insult, including wound debridement and treatment for exuberant hypergranulation tissue. After washing the wound, she recommended:

> . . . cotton sprinkled with aristol and smeared with a little ointment placed over it and kept in position with celloidin. For an abrasion, . . . painting with white of egg. . . . Another excellent dressing is a mixture of castor oil and bismuth. . . . The part is sponged clean with soft gauze sponges, a solution of boric acid or a weak solution of carbolic acid being employed, and the

[48]Higbee, "Practical Points," 336–338.
[49]Dorland, *American Medical Dictionary*, quote p. 95.
[50]Higbee, "Practical Points," 336–338, quote p. 337.

> cavity packed with strips of iodoform gauze or treated with iodoform or aristol ointment, over which a layer of borated cotton is applied. The whole is sealed with a layer of gauze wrapped in celloidin. . . . If there be slough, it may be removed . . . (by a) . . . packing of gauze moistened in carbolic solution. . . . Weak granulations may sometimes require stimulation: where they are too exuberant some caustic application may be indicated. . . .[51]

Charlotte Brown in the 1914 text *Junior Nurse* divided bedsores into two classes: one minor due to moisture and the other a more severe type, each with different treatment needs. She advocated removal of slough and keeping the minor lesion dry by ". . . applying a 4 per cent solution of boracic acid. The surface should be . . . powdered with an antiseptic powder. . . ."[52] However, moist healing was suggested when a more severe lesion was present. She stated:

> The treatment . . . consists of hot, moist dressings until the slough is removed, followed by one which will promote granulation, as fluffed gauze moistened with balsam of Peru, or equal parts alcohol, glycerin and tannin, loosely packed in.[53]

Stuart McGuire, in his 1915 surgical text, *The Profit and Loss Account of Modern Medicine and Other Papers*, identified the wide range of treatments available to treat bedsores, incorporating the concepts of antisepsis and infection prevention. In a chapter titled, "Methods to Hasten Epidermization," the selection of treatment modality was determined by wound characteristics and knowledge of wound healing:

> To secure epidermization the first step . . . stop suppuration . . . second . . . stimulate normal regeneration . . . protect the embryonal cells resulting . . . third, . . . augment nature's reparative forces by grafting the bare area with epithelial tissue of sufficient vitality not only to live, but to grow. . . . *Moist dressings*. . . . The cotton should be wet as soon as it becomes dry . . . changed as often as it becomes soiled. The solution . . . should not be a strong antiseptic, as it would kill cells as well as germs, but it should have an inhibitory action on microbic life. (solutions include) *chloral hydrate solution* . . .; *Thiersch's solution* . . .; and *acetate of aluminusolution*. . . . *Dry Dressings*. . . . powders most frequently iodoform, aristol, dermatol, bismuth, boric acid and oxide of zinc. *Oleaginous Dressings* . . . salves and ointments . . . has

---

[51]Hampton, *Nursing Principles and Practice*, 118–130, quote pp. 127–128.
[52]Brown, *Junior Nurse*, quote p. 94.
[53]Ibid., quote pp. 94–95.

> fallen into unmerited disfavor . . . Vaseline, lanoline and castor oil, plain or medicated, . . . exert a feeble antiseptic action, . . .; they exclude air, thus relieving pain; . . . prevent . . . adhesion of overlying dressings, thus saving the embryonal cells from mechanical injury. *Nutritive Dressings.* . . . dressing that supplies food directly to the germinal cells and their offspring. . . . Valentine's Meat Juice . . . is sterile, contains no alcohol, is rich in food stuff . . . applied on cotton in the form of a moist dressing. *Alterative Dressings.* . . . Nitrate of silver, mercurial ointment, chloride of zinc, and sulphate of copper . . . protonuclein. *Protective Dressings.* . . . Protection is best accomplished by interposing some impervious material between the granulations and the meshes of the overlying gauze, . . . Cargile membrane is made from the peritoneum of an ox . . . *Proliferating Dressing.* . . . When the destruction of skin is so extensive that the normal reparative power is insufficient to cover the granulating area. . . . [54]

Treatment based on wound characteristics resulted in different wound care practices. Georgiana Sanders, a nurse educator, described two classes of bedsores, those due to abrasion and those due to impaired circulation. She described skin injury consistent with deep tissue injury in bedsores caused by impaired circulation. In these bedsores, purple and bruised tissues deteriorate despite interventions, including removal of pressure. "Only rarely is it possible to avert a bed-sore once this bruised spot is noticed."[55] Once necrotic tissue develops in these wounds, debridement is recommended to aid healing:

> . . . at this stage . . . bathing with very hot water for ten minutes at a time, repeated hourly, painting the surface with the three tinctures (tincture of aconite. . ., tincture of opium. . ., tincture of iodine. . .) or strapping applied directly over the colored spot . . . (if a) slough has already formed, which must come away before healing can begin. . . . (Its removal) may be hastened by the application of hot compresses or a small poultice . . . covered, . . . with some moisture-proof protective, such as light mackintosh sheeting or gutta-percha tissue. . . .[56]

---

[54]Stuart McGuire, *The Profit and Loss Account of Modern Medicine and Other Papers* (Richmond, VA: L. H. Jenkins, 1915), quote pp. 265–269.

[55]Sanders, *Modern Methods*, quote p. 79. The National Pressure Ulcer Advisory Panel (NPUAP) added Suspected Deep Tissue Injury (DTI) to pressure ulcer staging system in 2007. DTI progresses from purple or maroon intact skin to large open wound quickly despite intervention. NPUAP, Pressure Ulcer Stages Revised by NPUAP: Updated Staging System. February 2007.

[56]Ibid., quote p. 80.

Sanders also described other wound characteristics and their appropriate treatment. Such wounds included an infected bedsore and a "stalled" wound in need of stimulation. Care for these various wounds included:

> . . . a sterile, mildly antiseptic dusting-powder constantly applied, such as starch and zinc, or stearate of zinc. . . . If the sore is progressing favorably, the surface will become clean and dry, and new granulations, in the form of bright red specks, may be observed . . . . in all wounds, there is consequently danger of infection . . . signs of such infection are discharge and local inflammation; the granulations are pale and unhealthy; the sore, instead of healing grows deep. . . . If stimulation is required, the surface is sometimes touched with nitrate of silver or blue stone, or an astringent lotion such as zinc wash, may be used.[57]

Large wounds according to Sanders also require different treatments including strict surgical asepsis and topical agents including peroxide of hydrogen, a bovinin, balsam of Peru, or a weak solution of zinc, known as red wash.[58]

Available treatments continued to evolve in the 1920s and 1930s, including the use of heat. While several treatments were in vogue from previous years, nurse Irene Kelly's recommendations included the use of a hot dressing and treatments such as stearate of zinc powder, castor, and zinc ointment alone or in combination, and the removal of necrotic tissue if present in the wound:

> . . . Cleanse (wound) . . . twice a day with equal parts of peroxide[e] of hydrogen and sterile water. . . . Then cleanse the part in same manner with boracic acid 2 per cent . . . apply a hot dressing of same. A dressing of Balsam of Peru may be substituted (for the hot boracic). . . .[59]

Pope and Young reiterated the need to rid the wound of slough and prevent infection in their 1935 text. However, they also advocated keeping the lesions dry to stimulate new tissues and healing, although others had promoted moist wound healing in the past.[60]

Later, in 1941, Mary Weston proposed a new method of wound care, demonstrating the advancement in the science and technology of bedsore treatment.[61] In this treatment protocol, rationales are given indicating the

---

[57]Ibid., 79.

[58]Ibid., 80.

[59]Kelley, *Text-Book of Nursing*, 1926: quote p. 43; 1936: quote p. 45.

[60]Pope and Young, *Art and Principles of Nursing*, 69–71

[61]Weston, "Paste Treatment," 388–390.

scientific basis of the treatment consisting of pastes applied to optimize the wound bed and promote moist wound healing and cell proliferation. The treatment protocol entailed the application of one of three pastes: pectin paste, tragacanth paste, and a urea (carbamide paste, progressively applied to the wound bed. A new paste was applied after the wound stopped responding to the previous one. Moreover, the choice of the paste was guided by wound cultures which identified organisms found in the wound.

CONCLUSION

Nurses have played a vital role in the development of knowledge related to pressure ulcers, wounds, and wound healing. In the first half of the twentieth century, this knowledge was in large part a result of informal trial and error at the bedside of the patients for whom they cared. Nursing texts served as a dominant vehicle for the dissemination of newfound nursing knowledge. Bedsores have remained a persistent problem for over a century. It is clear that nurses have known about bedsores and attempted to prevent them and cure them for over 100 years. It is also clear that we are battling the same foe—the same "obstinate . . . sore,"[62] as did our predecessors. Descriptions of pressure injury, sites of injury and sources of injury pressure, friction, and shear, facilitated by moisture, remain remarkably unchanged.

It is also clear that the debate over the avoidability of pressure ulcers and the culpability of nursing care in their development has also continued for over a century. One is also left to ponder . . . is it likely that for over a century, nurses would allow a bedsore to occur if it was at all within his or her capabilities to prevent its occurrence and attendant suffering?

---

[62]Dorland, *American Medical Dictionary*, quote p. 95.

Section II

NURSING INTERVENTIONS: OFFERING SERVICE

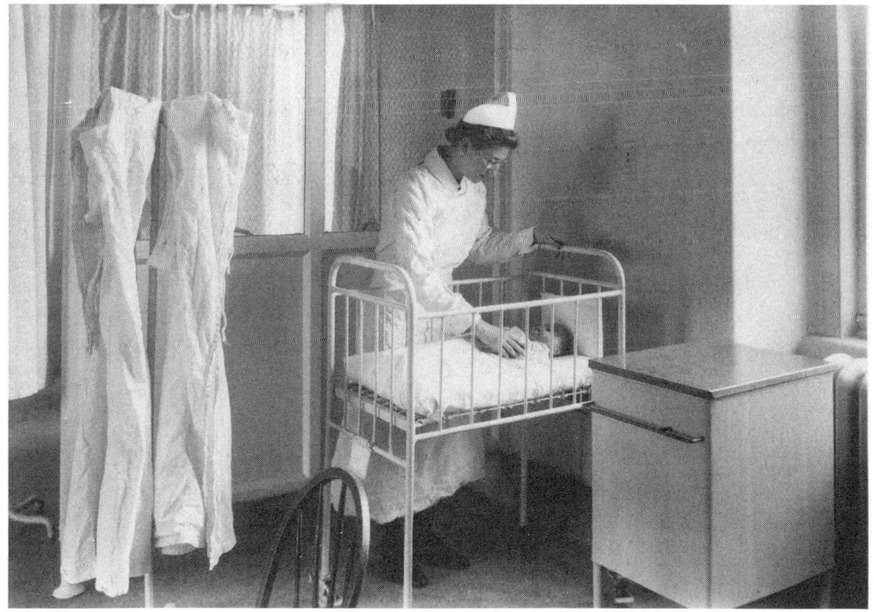

Student Nurse at Philadelphia General Hospital Using Semi-Isolation Technique in a Teaching Unit for Infant Care, ca. 1930s. *Reprinted with permission of the Barbara Bates Center for the Study of the History of Nursing.*

CHAPTER 5

Body, Soul, and Service: Catholic Sister-Nurses in Late Nineteenth and Early Twentieth Century Hospitals

Barbra Mann Wall

INTRODUCTION

On Monday, January 1, 1900, the Sisters of Charity of the Incarnate Word admitted Mrs. S. W.,[1] a private patient, to Santa Rosa Infirmary in San Antonio, Texas. S. W. remained in the company of a sister-nurse, who stayed with her throughout the night. The next morning, in an operating room that had been constructed 4 years earlier, Dr. A. S. McDaniel performed a hysterectomy on S. W. Dr. McDaniel was a prominent surgeon in San Antonio, having received his training in both the United States and Europe. According to the sisters' hospital chronicles, the "operation went well, and [she] is doing nicely."[2] Three weeks later, on January 22, she was discharged. Because her stay at Santa Rosa included the first Friday of the month, S. W. would have had an opportunity to participate in a devotion the sisters held in their hospital chapel. This devotion was the exposition of the Blessed Sacrament, whereby the "consecrated host" was

[1]For confidentiality reasons, the patient's name has been changed.

[2]*Remark Book, Santa Rosa Infirmary* (hereafter cited as *RBSR*), January 1 and 2, 1900, Archives of the Motherhouse of the Incarnate Word, San Antonio, Texas (hereafter cited as AMIW).

displayed for the faithful to observe and worship.[3] That particular month, the sisters held it all day Friday until 7:30 P.M. and again on Sunday until 3:00 P.M.[4]

In this chapter, case histories from three Catholic nursing orders are examined: the Sisters of St. Joseph of Carondelet from St. Paul, Minnesota; the Sisters of Charity of the Incarnate Word from San Antonio, Texas; and the Sisters of the Holy Cross from South Bend, Indiana. Many were immigrants from Ireland, Germany, and France. Between 1865 and 1920, these congregations operated and owned more than 40 general, miners', marine, and railroad hospitals in the West and Midwest.[5] In the context of nineteenth- and twentieth-century immigration and social upheaval, sisters constructed both medical and sacred space within the environment of the hospital. To understand the contemporary conception of nursing as caring for the whole person—body, mind, and spirit—we can turn to an historical narrative of sister-nurses' practices that demonstrates performance of physical, psychological, and spiritual care.

Despite our tendency to see science and religion as mutually exclusive, Catholic sister-nurses' experiences suggest that this was not historically the case. Their hospitals were, first, expressions of religious and charitable principles. Catholic tradition guided their works, in particular rituals and symbols, and in their own presence with patients. At the same time, nuns blended their religious activities and nursing practices with scientific medicine to provide greater access to diagnosis and care of the sick and dying.

CATHOLIC HOSPITAL ESTABLISHMENT, 1849–1911

Between 1866 and 1926, nuns established nearly 500 healthcare institutions in the United States.[6] Like secular hospitals, Catholic hospitals of the early

---

[3]Devotions were expressions of popular piety. See Richard P. McBrien, ed., *The Harper Collins Encyclopedia of Catholicism* (San Francisco, CA: Harper Collins Publishers, 1989), 504. Ann Taves asserts, "Veneration of the Blessed Sacrament was a devotional reflection of the Catholic doctrine of the real presence" of Christ. See Ann Taves, *The Household of Faith: Roman Catholic Devotions in Mid-Nineteenth Century America* (Notre Dame, IN: University of Notre Dame Press, 1986), 30. She uses the image of "the household of faith" to describe the familial-like relationships between Catholics and saints.

[4]*RBSR*, January 5 and 7, 1900, AMIW.

[5]Barbra Mann Wall, *Unlikely Entrepreneurs: Catholic Sisters and the Hospital Marketplace, 1865–1925* (Columbus, OH: Ohio State University Press, 2005).

[6]John O'Grady, *Catholic Charities in the United States: History and Problems* (Washington, DC: National Conference of Catholic Charities, 1930), 195–196; "The Chronological

twentieth century changed from primarily charitable institutions to modern medical facilities that focused on curative services and surgical intervention for an expanding number of privately paying patients. Sisters adapted to the secular and scientific advances, but moderated these trends to allow their hospitals to function as both medical and religious institutions.

Several issues were at stake for Catholics. Immigration had more than doubled the total number of Catholics in the United States by 1860, and even larger increases occurred after 1890.[7] By then, Catholic immigration rates were growing faster than those of other denominations, especially in cities. While Protestant growth occurred particularly in the southern regions of the country, Catholic enclaves of European immigrants predominated in Eastern cities such as New York, Boston, and Philadelphia, and Midwestern cities such as St. Paul, St. Louis, and Chicago. Immigrants from Mexico helped San Antonio's Catholic population grow as well. The Catholic Church was in the minority in Utah and parts of Texas, but these states attracted many immigrant miners and railroad workers from Catholic countries who were potential American Catholics. Church leaders sensed that significant Catholic populations existed with inadequate spiritual institutions. To tap the immigrant populations and counteract Protestant proselytizing, the Catholic Church created separate institutions and defined them along religious lines. Leaders sought religious women to staff these facilities, in which they could preserve the Catholic identity.[8]

Table 5.1 shows the hospitals established by the three congregations represented in this chapter. The Congregation of the Sisters of St. Joseph

---

Development of the Catholic Hospital in the United States and Canada," *Hospital Progress* 21 (April 1940), 122–133; Ursula Stepsis and Dolores Liptak, eds., *Pioneer Healers: The History of Women Religious in American Health Care* (New York: Crossroad, 1989), 287. Male religious orders such as the Alexian Brothers also have a long history of hospital establishment.

[7]Jay P. Dolan, *The American Catholic Experience: A History From Colonial Times to the Present* (Notre Dame, IN: University of Notre Dame Press, 1992), 127–157; William Peterson, Michael Novak, and Philip Gleason, *Concepts of Ethnicity* (Cambridge, MA: Belknap Press of Harvard University Press, 1982), 69; Roger Finke and Rodney Stark, *The Churching of America, 1776–1990: Winners and Losers in Our Religious Economy* (New Brunswick, NJ: Rutgers University Press, 1992), 109–144.

[8]Dolan, *American Catholic Experience*, 127–157; Jay P. Dolan, *The Immigrant Church: New York's Irish and German Catholics, 1815-1865* (Baltimore, MD: Johns Hopkins University Press, 1975).

TABLE 5.1 Selected Catholic Hospital Development, 1849–1911

Congregation	Hospital site	Date of establishment
Sisters of St. Joseph of Carondelet		
	Philadelphia, PA	1849
	Wheeling, [West] VA	1853
	St. Paul, MN	1854
	Kansas City, MO	1874
	Prescott, AZ	1878
	Georgetown, CO	1880
	Tucson, AZ	1880
	Keshena, WI	1886
	Minneapolis, MN	1887
	Hancock, MI	1889
	Fargo, ND	1900
	Amsterdam, NY	1903
	Grand Forks, ND	1907
	Troy, NY	1908
Sisters of the Holy Cross		
	Cairo, IL	1867
	Salt Lake City, UT	1875
	Deadwood, Dakota Terr.	1878
	Silver Reef, UT	1879
	Columbus, OH	1886
	South Bend, IN	1889
Sisters of Charity of the Incarnate Word		
	San Antonio, TX	1869
	Marshall, TX	1885
	Ft. Worth, TX	1889
	Boerne, TX	1896
	Amarillo, TX	1901
	St. Louis, MO	1902
	Corpus Christie, TX	1905
	San Angelo, TX	1910
	Paris, TX	1911

From Sister Margaret Patrice Slattery, CCVI, "Historical Studies of Hospitals"; Savage, *The Congregation of St. Joseph of Carondelet*, 100–102; Congregation of the Sisters of the Holy Cross Establishments, 1843–1971.

of Carondelet was one of the earliest European women's religious communities to work in hospitals in the United States. Between 1849 and 1908, these women established 14 hospitals in all parts of the country. They also nursed in both the Civil War and the Spanish-American War.[9] After the Civil War, the Sisters of the Holy Cross and the Sisters of Charity of the Incarnate Word became involved in healthcare. These congregations were particularly active in the West, Midwest, and Southwest as they followed the immigrants into new industrial, railroad, and mining centers. As they had done in the Civil War, the Sisters of the Holy Cross also volunteered their nursing during the Spanish-American War.[10] The Congregation of the Sisters of Charity of the Incarnate Word was founded specifically to meet healthcare needs in Texas. These sisters opened general hospitals, homes for the aged and mentally ill, and rehabilitation facilities. By 1911, in addition to nine general hospitals listed in Table 5.1, the Incarnate Word Sisters directed six other railroad hospitals in Tyler and Palestine, Texas; in Las Vegas, New Mexico; in Fort Madison, Iowa; and in Sedalia and Kansas City, Missouri.[11]

Catholic hospitals in the United States developed under a variety of circumstances. They evolved in response to medical and nursing needs of local and regional communities resulting from epidemics, wars, and industrial injuries. They also grew from general institutions for the indigent and provided multifaceted services for the sick poor, widows, the aged, and children. Unlike Protestant institutions, Catholic hospitals in the United States were not primarily started to provide wealthy benefactors a means of patronage. While some collaborative teaching ventures between Catholic sisters and medical schools existed, a Catholic hospital's primary purpose was to heal

---

[9]Barbra Mann Wall, "'Called to a Mission of Charity': The Sisters of St. Joseph in the Civil War," *Nursing History Review* 6 (1998): 85–113; Dolorita Marie Dougherty, et al., *Sisters of St. Joseph of Carondelet* (St. Louis, MO: B. Herder Book Co., 1966), 368; Carol K. Coburn and Martha Smith, "'Pray for Your Wanderers': Women Religious on the Colorado Mining Frontier, 1877–1917," *Frontiers* 15 (1995): 27–52; Carol K. Coburn and Martha Smith, *Spirited Lives: How Nuns Shaped Catholic Culture and American Life, 1836–1920* (Chapel Hill, NC: University of North Carolina Press, 1999), 190–191; Mary Lucinda Savage, *The Congregation of St. Joseph of Carondelet: A Brief Account of Its Origin and Its Work in the United States, 1650–1922* (St. Louis, MO: Herder Book, Col, 1923), 100–102.

[10]Congregation of the Sisters of the Holy Cross Establishments, 1843–1971, Archives of the Congregation of the Sisters of the Holy Cross, Saint Mary's, Notre Dame, Indiana (hereafter cited as CSC). See also Barbra Mann Wall, "Grace under Pressure: The Nursing Sisters of the Holy Cross, 1861–1865," *Nursing History Review* 1 (1993): 71–97; Barbra Mann Wall, "Courage to Care: The Sisters of the Holy Cross in the Spanish-American War," *Nursing History Review* 3 (1995): 55–77.

[11]Sister Margaret Patrice Slattery, CCVI, "Historical Studies of Hospitals, Schools in Mexico, and Incarnate Word College," in *Promises to Keep: A History of the Sisters of Charity of the Incarnate Word, San Antonio, Texas*, vol. 2 (San Antonio, TX: private printing, 1995).

and comfort the infirm, the sick, and the dying and to afford them the opportunity for repentance and spiritual solace.[12]

SPIRITUAL AGENTS OF CARE

As they modernized their hospitals and their nursing practices to accommodate technical advances of medical science, sisters also expanded the "sacred space" in their facilities.[13] One way was by building new hospital chapels. Because sacraments were important, chapels were necessary for any Catholic institutions that sheltered the sick and dying. Nurses and patients assembled there to pray and to attend religious services such as Mass. In 1883 in Salt Lake City, a newspaper article described Holy Cross Hospital's chapel as "a perfect gem of its kind."[14] Chapels were close to patients' rooms or wards so that those who were unable to walk could have their beds moved into nearby hallways and participate in Mass. At St. Mary's, Minneapolis, for example, patients on the third floor south wing could see the chapel's altar. A Catholic bulletin reflected the integration of science and religion in Catholic hospitals: "Secular hospitals and sanatoria may embody in their structure and equipment, even as does St. Mary's, the latest and best ideas of the scientific builder," but only Catholic hospitals had chapels "wherein abides the Author of life and the Hope of those who die."[15] Sisters dealt with the tensions between medical and sacred space by locating their chapels away from operating rooms and other areas that required more rigorous attention to germ-free environments.

---

[12]The first hospital staffed by the Daughters of Charity in the continental United States in 1823 was the Baltimore Infirmary, a teaching hospital. Collaborative teaching ventures between sisters and medical schools also existed in places such as Georgetown University and the Mayo Clinic. See Alma S. Woolley, *Learning, Faith, And Caring: History of the Georgetown University School of Nursing, 1903–2000* (private printing, 2001); Sioban Nelson, *Say Little, Do Much: Nursing, Nuns, and Hospitals in the Nineteenth Century* (Philadelphia, PA: University of Pennsylvania Press, 2001), 45–47. See also Christopher J. Kauffman, *Ministry and Meaning: A Religious History of Catholic Health Care in the United States* (New York: Crossroad Publishing, 1995).

[13]"Sacred space" is discussed in Mircea Eliade, *The Sacred and the Profane: The Nature of Religion* (New York: Harcourt, Brace and World, 1959), 20–65. Ellen Skerrett has used the term in "Creating Sacred Space in an Early Chicago Neighborhood," in *At the Crossroads: Old Saint Patrick's and the Chicago Irish*, ed. Ellen Skerrett (Chicago, IL: Loyola Press and Wild Onion Books, 1997), 21–38. See also Taves, *Household of Faith*, 122.

[14]*Salt Lake Tribune*, June 3, 1883.

[15]"St. Mary's New Hospital," *Catholic Bulletin*, September 7, 1918.

Many chapels were quite large and could seat up to 200 people. Indeed, these large basilicas underline the point that these hospitals were Catholic edifices. They were emblems of Church power, piety, and selflessness. Holy Cross Hospital's large chapel in Salt Lake City, a Mormon bastion, surely embodied a major statement by the Catholic Church.

Although they integrated the scientific fashions of the times, Catholic hospitals' central justification was to bring the hope of Christ's healing and salvation to patients.[16] Belief in miraculous healings was common for Roman Catholics throughout the nineteenth and early twentieth centuries. This involved belief in the supernatural power of religious objects. Relics were particularly popular.[17] At the opening of a new wing at St. Joseph's Hospital in South Bend, Indiana, the Sisters of the Holy Cross and local Catholic leaders put symbolic items in the cornerstone that included relics of 10 saints, which officials then placed beneath a 9-foot-high Celtic cross on top of the building.[18] Nuns also kept shrines, statues, pictures of saints, fonts of holy water, and crucifixes in patients' rooms and hospital corridors. For example, a private room at St. Paul's St. Joseph's Hospital in the early 1900s featured leather-upholstered chairs, a brass bed, a stained-glass window, and a small Marian statue on the wall.[19] Sisters used beads, scapulars, medals, prayer books, and holy pictures to heal or at least to lead a suffering person closer to God. Their understanding of the importance of the supernatural power of relics, medals, and holy water for restoring and safeguarding individuals could help Catholic patients facing death or undergoing other medical crises. A small but significant part of hospital budgets included religious vessels, ornaments, and chapel expenses.[20]

Nuns also dedicated their hospitals to patron saints. When the Incarnate Word Sisters purchased the Missouri Pacific Railroad Hospital in Fort Worth, Texas, they immediately changed the name to St. Joseph's, the patron saint of the Catholic Church.[21] They also renovated the building to reflect their

---

[16]Kauffman, *Ministry and Meaning*, 145.

[17]Dolan, *American Catholic Experience*, 234.

[18]"Corner Stone Laid," *South Bend Tribune*, April 27, 1903. In PINS 020/03, University of Notre Dame Archives, Notre Dame, Indiana.

[19]Fifty-Eighth Report of St. Joseph's Hospital, St. Paul, Minnesota, Archives of the Congregation of the Sisters of St. Joseph of Carondelet, St. Paul Province, St. Paul, Minnesota (hereafter cited as ACSJC-SP), 300.2-1, box 2, folder 10.

[20]For example, see "Annual Account for 1 July 1914 to 1 July 1915," *Holy Cross Hospital Budgets and Accounts, 1892-July 1941*; "Cost of 1902 Building, Holy Cross Hospital," CSC; "Financial Reports of St. Mary's Hospital, ACSJC-SP.

[21]Pius IX declared St. Joseph as the patron of the Catholic Church in 1870, and devotions to St. Joseph were frequent thereafter. See Taves, *Household of Faith*, 39; McBrien, *Encyclopedia*, 718–719.

Catholicism. A priest blessed each room in the hospital, the stables, and the outdoor buildings and nailed holy medals to infirmary doors. The motherhouse in San Antonio sent crucifixes, fonts, saints' statues, and water that a priest had blessed.[22] Four stained-glass panels in the chapel window incorporated several symbols of Christ. Together, they conveyed the message that Christ delivered the faithful from sin and death.[23]

Catholic tradition was also evident in the sisters' own presence with patients, which could be a sign to others of a dimension beyond the visible world of everyday experiences.[24] Sisters' comforting, feeding, and sheltering the sick and dying, and their whispers of consoling prayers to patients in pain or near death functioned as invitations to religious experiences and means for patients to meet God. To convey the message that they wished to relate to others on a deeper, more spiritual level, sisters consistently underscored their "asexual" identities, not merely by their vow of chastity but also through their religious dress, which concealed their physical bodies. Symbolic of their "purity of intention," to serve God in the person of the sick, nuns wore crucifixes, hearts, and rosaries.[25]

In the early decades of the twentieth century, sisters adapted their clothing to meet newer scientific standards. In November of 1897, Incarnate Word Sisters at Santa Rosa Infirmary wore white veils for the first time during an operation, and had white caps made for the doctors.[26] A nun who entered training in 1910 at St. Joseph's, St. Paul, became a surgical nurse and designed her own uniform: she pinned up her black skirt and sleeves under a white doctor's gown and wore a white outer veil over the black one.[27] For many sisters, a change in habit did not come about until after 1915 in response to the hospital standardization movement. Discussion at that time centered around sisters' wearing white washable habits while on duty instead of black woolen ones, which, in the eyes of some medical authorities, harbored germs. Some conservative religious leaders opposed any change in sisters' habits because they feared it would compromise nuns' religious identities.[28] Nonetheless, sisters maintained their religious identities by wearing veils with other symbols such as crosses.

---

[22]*Remark Book, St. Joseph's Hospital* (hereafter cited as *RBSJ*), April 23 and 24, 1889, AMIW.
[23]See F. R. Webber, *Church Symbolism* (Cleveland, OH: J.H. Jansen, 1938), 57–65; D. Apostolos-Cappodona, *Dictionary of Christian Art* (New York: Continuum, 1994), 91, 203–204, 275.
[24]Joseph Marcos, *Doors to the Sacred: A Historical Introduction to the Sacraments in the Catholic Church* (Liguori, MO: Triumph Books, 1991), 393.
[25]Kauffman, *Ministry and Meaning*, 212.
[26]*RBSR*, November 20, 1897, AMIW.
[27]Sister Ann Joachim Moore, "History of the School of Nursing, St. Mary's Hospital," 1957, 14, ACSJC-SP.
[28]Kauffman, *Ministry and Meaning*, 181–183.

Several written documents provide insight into the training and nursing practice of Catholic sister-nurses. They cared for people of all religious faiths, particularly in the western mining camps where religious diversity was especially prominent. Sisters' constitutions articulated how they were to care for the sick, what daily schedule nurses should follow, how they should relate to physicians, how they were to prepare food and medicines, and by what means the sisters should prepare a person for death. Nuns were to speak softly and to work gently, quietly, and unhurriedly. Most patients until the twentieth century were males, and nuns tried to obtain male nurses to help with them. As far as can be determined from the records, however, there were not enough to make it possible to enforce this rule. Thus, directives also emphasized the need for modesty.[29] Prescriptions also focused on compassionate attitudes for sister-nurses. The Incarnate Word Sisters were to "serve [patients] with a tireless zeal," and "entertain for the sick, not only a compassion, kindness and devotedness, but likewise a great respect." The Sisters of the Holy Cross were to be mild, vigilant, patient yet firm, and compassionate for the suffering of others.[30]

At the same time, nuns' nursing practices conveyed a distinct religious vision. The sisters' constitutions had specific guidelines for Catholic patients: Nuns were to effect changes not only in a sick person's physical health but also in his or her religious attitudes and behaviors through provision of religious instruction and guidance. While sister-nurses were to follow the doctor's orders for medications and physical care, they also were to exhort the sick and dying Catholic or potential Catholic patient to penance, resignation, and prayer. For Protestants, however, the rules were different. The Sisters of St. Joseph were to respect Protestants' religious convictions and show them "the greatest courtesy and kindness."[31] Likewise, the Incarnate Word Sisters were "by no means" to "advance their opinion and religious beliefs" to non-Catholics. If they thought someone was in physical or spiritual danger, they were to "guide them toward the mercy of God," but they should "never have a debate with anybody in regard to matters of faith."[32]

Sisters' very work, however, was a powerful form of evangelism. They proselytized by the virtue of their deeds and accomplished conversions in this way. For example, when Sister Augusta Anderson went to Utah in 1875, she wrote to her priest superior that the best way to do any good with the

---

[29]For further discussion on this topic, see Sioban Nelson, "Reading Nursing History," *Nursing Inquiry* 4 (1997): 229–236.

[30]See *Directory of the Sisters of Charity of the Incarnate Word*, 1906, 207, AMIW; *Rules of the Congregation of the Sisters of the Holy Cross*, 1895, 142, CSC.

[31]*Manual of Decrees*, 114, ACSJC-St. Louis Province (hereafter cited as ACSJC-SL).

[32]*1873 Directory* (of the Sisters of Charity of the Incarnate Word), 5–6, AMIW.

Mormons is "to have little to say, and give them good example."[33] In 1898, soon after the Sisters of the Holy Cross arrived at Camp Hamilton during the Spanish-American War, Mother Annunciata McSheffery instructed them to avoid preaching to the sick men, but, instead, to exercise "the eloquent silence of prayer and good example. This is the best method of doing good."[34] Sometimes, however, proselytizing methods could be subtle. During the Spanish-American War, for example, the Sisters of St. Joseph shared scapulars, crucifixes, medals, and beads with Catholic soldiers. As they did, they were conscious of non-Catholics in nearby beds who were listening to what they said. As a result, Sister Liguori McNamara could write that both Catholic and Protestant soldiers asked for medals.[35] Some non-Catholics asked to join the Catholic Church as they neared death.

Sisters' nursing practices were particularly important in a religion such as Catholicism that emphasized ritual. For Catholics, the central rituals were the Mass and sacraments. Thus, nuns often accompanied patients to Mass in hospital chapels. They also incorporated various healing practices associated not only with regular medicine but also with devotions. These included devotions to the saints and the Virgin Mary, who, Catholics believed, had power over disease. During the nineteenth century, the Catholic Church revived other exercises, such as the rosary, the 40-hour devotion, benediction, and devotions to the Sacred Heart and the Immaculate Conception. Associated with saints were novenas, or 9-day devotions to honor a saint or make a particular request.[36] Although they did not require participation of non-Catholic patients, sister-nurses promoted elaborate religious ceremonies in their hospitals. At the Incarnate Word Sisters' hospitals, both nuns and patients celebrated religious feasts, held 40 hours of adoration in chapels, and processed in hallways and on hospital grounds.[37]

Sisters also prayed with their patients. Catholic belief held that prayer, along with the sacraments, brought grace and favors from Jesus and Mary, including cure of the sick. Lay Catholics often asked sisters to pray for them, believing that nuns' prayers were more powerful than their own. In 1897, a patient requested his remaining salary to go to the Sisters of Charity of the

---

[33]Sister Augusta Anderson to Father Sorin, July 13, 1875, CSC.

[34]Mother M. Annunciata McSheffery, *Circular Letter to Sisters*, September 9, 1898, CSC.

[35]Sister Liguori to Reverend Mother, October 31, and December 1, 1898, ACSJC-SL.

[36]Dolan, *American Catholic Experience*, 229–233; Taves, *Household of Faith*, 30. The 40-hours devotion focused on the Blessed Sacrament and involved a period of 40 hours' adoration, depicting the 40 hours that Jesus's body was in the sepulcher.

[37]*RBSJ*, March 25, 1892; *RBSR*, February 17 and August 15, 1896; January 18 and February 20, 1898, AMIW.

Incarnate Word at Santa Rosa Infirmary in return for their prayers after he died. A few months later, family members removed a woman's remains from one cemetery to another that was closer to Santa Rosa so the Incarnate Word Sisters would pray for her when they visited the site.[38] In addition to healing the sick, one of the corporal works of mercy, according to Catholic tradition, was to bury the dead.[39] The Incarnate Word Sisters kept a "dead house" behind Santa Rosa Infirmary, which held bodies of the deceased until relatives arrived. Sisters frequently held wakes in their hospital parlors, and families often asked nuns to attend to burial services.[40]

Caring for the dying was particularly important to Catholic sisters. In the late nineteenth century, most patients died at home, but Catholic writers asserted that a Catholic hospital was the most appropriate place for their parishioners to die.[41] Here, sister-nurses hoped to strengthen the sick or dying person's soul and help him or her more easily bear illness and resist temptations. In Catholic hospitals, patients could receive not only physical care grounded in science but also the sacraments. Catholic theology held that grace, which the sacraments conferred, could save the soul of the dying. Thus, to die in a state of grace, it was absolutely necessary for a person to have opportunities to make a last confession and receive the sacraments. The three most important sacraments for the sick person were Anointing the Sick, the Eucharist (or Holy Communion), and Baptism.[42] While sisters could not administer the first two, they could baptize a patient in the absence of a priest. Most important, they would be present to call priests and thus see that these important deathbed rituals were carried out.

Yet, sister-nurses' experiences were not homogeneous. The politics of some states made it incautious to openly evangelize. Many hospitals in New York, for example, were funded by the state, and to prevent any controversy, sisters meticulously avoided any proselytizing and welcomed both Catholic and non-Catholic clergy in their hospitals.[43]

Historian Robert Orsi accurately depicted sister nurses' work when he asserted that, when they "brought the Virgin and saints into hospitals and sickrooms," they "were not merely complementing the sacramental work of

---

[38]*RBSR*, January 6 and October 27, 1897, AMIW.

[39]McBrien, *Encyclopedia*, 854.

[40]Slattery, *Promises to Keep*, 213; *RBSR*, October 24, 1896, AMIW.

[41]Thomas Dwight, "The Training Schools for Nurses of the Sisters of Charity," *Catholic World* 61 (May 1895): 191.

[42]McBrien, *Encyclopedia*, 146–147.

[43]Barbra Mann Wall and Sioban Nelson, "'Our Heels Are Praying Very Hard All Day'," *Holistic Nursing Practice* 17, no. 6 (November–December 2003): 320–328.

the clergy (or the medical efforts of the physician)." As they said rosaries, made novenas, accompanied patients to Mass in their chapels, and maintained hospital shrines, they conveyed "an alternative understanding of what was possible for the ill, medically and religiously, in the spaces of the hospital and sickroom."[44] Indeed, these devotional practices subtly undermined male physicians' authority with their narrowly focused medical goals.[45]

BOTH SCIENTIFIC AND RELIGIOUS NURSING PRACTICES

In the late nineteenth and early twentieth centuries, the sisters were part of a Catholic tradition still trying to earn respectability. Thus, their annual reports highlighted to physicians and prospective patients that hospital personnel would practice scientific medicine. These publications showed an integration of science and religion, with photographs of sisters in their religious habits working in areas such as sterile operating rooms. It was their attempt to present themselves as scientific and professional.[46] Indeed, by 1920, sisters had accepted much of the redefinition of hospital care and nursing that began in the late nineteenth century with the rise of science-intensive medicine. Yet they also incorporated this redefinition into a concept of hospital care that remained distinctly religious. This was due, in large part, to the sisters' own commanding presence and their special gender and religious identities. Their nursing practices incorporated scientific principles along with religious rituals, devotions, evangelism, and the sacraments. Catholic hospital architecture also reflected a sacred atmosphere for patients, with chapels, crucifixes, and other religious icons.

One must be cautious in concluding that all of the sisters' religious nursing practices were sensitive to patient's needs. Nightingale herself disparaged some Catholic sisters in the Crimea because, to her, they were more interested in preparing patients for death than restoring them to life. In her *Notes on Nursing*, she charged that European sisters neglected their patients' general conditions, and she accused them of allowing a patient to "die of a bedsore, because the nurse may spread the dressing for it, but must not look at it."[47] In addition, the

---

[44]Robert A. Orsi, *Thank You, St. Jude: Women's Devotion to the Patron Saint of Hopeless Causes* (New Haven, CT: Yale University Press, 1996), 167.

[45]Ibid.

[46]Wall, *Unlikely Entrepreneurs*.

[47]Florence Nightingale, *Notes on Nursing* (New York: D. Appletonand Company; 1860; repr. London: Longman, Green and Roberts, 1969), 184. Here, Nightingale was decrying some European sisters' practices of not "looking" at wounds, which they viewed would contradict their vow of chastity.

evangelical nature of sisters' work likely offended some patients. Still, religion appealed to others who knew they were about to die and render an account of their lives. By helping patients express their beliefs, by facilitating important rituals and sacraments, and by staying with patients during their illness, sisters provided for spiritual needs. And for many patients, when they entered Catholic hospitals and observed a seamless integration of technology and spirituality, they were subtly given assurance that they were not only in the care of skilled professionals but also in the hands of the Divine.

ACKNOWLEDGMENTS

This chapter has been taken from the author's "Science and Ritual: The Hospital as Medical and Sacred Space, 1865–1920," *Nursing History Review* 11 (2003): 51–68.

The author thanks the Sisters of the Holy Cross in Notre Dame, Indiana; the Sisters of Charity of the Incarnate Word in San Antonio, Texas; and the Sisters of St. Joseph of Carondelet in St. Paul, Minnesota, for permission to use their collections. The author also thanks the University of Notre Dame and Purdue University for providing funding for this research.

SUGGESTIONS FOR FURTHER READING

Catherine A. Brekus, ed., *The Religious History of American Women: Reimagining the Past.* Chapel Hill, NC: University of North Carolina Press, 2007.

Patricia D'Antonio, "Nurses, Wives, and Mothers: Women and the Latter-Day Saints Training School's Class of 1919," *Journal of Women's History* 19, no. 3 (2007): 112–136.

Bernadette McCauley, *Who Shall Take Care of Our Sick? Roman Catholic Sisters and the Development of Catholic Hospitals in New York City*. Baltimore, MD: Johns Hopkins University Press, 2005.

Colleen McDannell, *Material Christianity: Religion and Popular Culture in America.* New Haven, CT: Yale University Press, 1995.

Sioban Nelson, *Say Little, Do Much: Nursing, Nuns, and Hospitals in the Nineteenth Century.* Philadelphia, PA: University of Pennsylvania Press, 2001.

James, M. O'Toole, ed., *Habits of Devotion: Catholic Religious Practice in Twentieth-Century America.* Ithaca, NY: Cornell University Press, 2004.

Barbra Mann Wall, "Religion and Gender in a Men's Hospital and School of Nursing, 1866–1969," *Nursing Research* 58, no. 3 (May/June 2009): 158–165.

Barbra Mann Wall, *Unlikely Entrepreneurs: Catholic Sisters and the Hospital Marketplace, 1865–1925*. Columbus, OH: Ohio State University Press, 2005.

Barbra Mann Wall and Sioban Nelson, "Our Heels Are Praying Very Hard All Day," *Holistic Nursing Practice* 17, no. 6 (November–December 2003): 320–328.

CHAPTER 6

Bridging the Gaps: Collaborative Health Work in the City of Brotherly Love, 1900–1920

J. Margo Brooks Carthon

INTRODUCTION

A major heart attack in the fellowship hall of a predominately African American church in Philadelphia prompted a group of health professionals belonging to the congregation to form a "Health Commission" to address excessive illness in the community. Church member and registered nurse Renee Cook was present during the unexpected health emergency and was among the first to respond to the crisis. She, along with the Health Commission's board of directors (comprising physicians, personal trainers, and nutritionists), hosted a day of free screenings and educational dialog during the summer of 2008. The mini-health fair was open to church members and community residents and was designed to combat high rates of heart disease among African Americans by increasing hypertension awareness and weight loss. Participants were offered free blood pressure screenings, interactive workshops on exercise, classes on healthy food preparation, and gardening tips.[1]

[1]Harold Brubaker, "Historic Church Holds Health Fair," available at: http://www.nursing.upenn.edu/media/Documents/Lewis%20Inquirer.pdf (accessed August 19, 2009).

This example of a grassroots health promotion effort in a Philadelphia church offers a contemporary example of nurses and other professionals working collectively to address the pressing health concerns of a local minority community. Nurses who are actively engaged in such collaborative efforts are well prepared by position and education to help promote health among populations at high risk for illness. Despite a long history of offering healthcare in community settings, questions remain on the best measures to ensure participation from community members on desired health initiatives: Must healthcare providers be of the same racial or ethnic group to ensure the success of health promotion efforts? And who should initiate health activities: health professionals or community residents themselves?

The case study presented in this chapter returns to early twentieth-century Philadelphia in search of clues to solving this dilemma by examining the successes of a health campaign from an earlier period. It begins with a description of the social environment and health status of Black Philadelphians living in South Philadelphia, and then moves to the collaborative campaign spearheaded by nurses to promote health in the community. It concludes with a discussion on the importance of building strong ties between nurses and community members in order to promote neighborhood-oriented health interventions.

THE PHYSICAL AND SOCIAL ENVIRONMENT OF BLACKS IN EARLY TWENTIETH-CENTURY PHILADELPHIA

At the opening of the twentieth century, Philadelphia was one of the oldest cities in the nation and was quickly becoming one of the most industrialized. Its growing manufacturing industry and rail lines made it an attractive destination to large numbers of Black southern migrants who entered the city in the decades following the Civil War in search of jobs and increased social freedom.[2] During the first 3 years of the century, the size of Philadelphia's black community more than tripled from 64,206 in 1900

[2]Allen F. Davis, *The Peoples of Philadelphia: A History of Ethnic Groups and Lower Class Life, 1790–1940* (Philadlephia, PA: Temple University Press, 1973), 7–10; Roger Lane, *Roots of Vilence in Black Philadelphia, 1860–1900* (Cambridge, MA: Harvard University Press), 1986.

to 219,559 in 1930.[3] By 1930, Philadelphia held the largest proportion of blacks in the country second only to Baltimore.[4]

Upon entering the city, many blacks faced economic hardships, excessive illness, and a severe housing shortage. The scarcity in housing was magnified due to overt practices of housing discrimination, which forced blacks to find housing in already cramped quarters of the city.[5] When housing was available, blacks were frequently charged higher rents. Faced with few choices, many migrant families crammed into dwellings that were meant to house only one.[6] Census figures for 1900 reveal that there were more than 4,000 single-unit homes in the city occupied by three or more families, very few of which were originally built for this purpose and without the benefit of structural modifications.[7] Many of the homes suffered from insufficient toileting, sewage, and water supply. If indoor toileting was available, up to four or five families shared a single water closet meant to serve only one. These water closets were regarded as particularly unsanitary: They frequently leaked, became obstructed, and in many instances overflowed, and in winter months, they often froze.[8] As many as 95% of blacks rented their homes, which left the responsibility of repairs to slumlords who were loathe to make them.

---

[3]Sadie T. Mossell, "The Standard of Living among One Hundred Negro Migrant Families in Philadelphia," *Annals of the American Academy of Political and Social Science* 98 (November 1921): 174–175. For more on the changes in Philadelphia's Black population and the assimilation of Blacks into the industiral working class, see Armstrong Association, "Report of Negro Population and Industries in Philadelphia," mimeographed manuscript, Armstron Association Papers, Temple Urban Archive (Philadelphia, PA, 1927).

[4]Henry R. M. Landis, *A Report of the Tuberculosis Problem and the Negro* (Philadelphia, PA: Henry Phipps Institute, 1923): Table 2, page 4, and Table 6, titled: *Showing the Composition of the Population of Seven Large Cities in the United States in 1920, with Particular Reference to the Negro Component.*

[5]Booker T. Washington, "Letter to the Editor," *Philadelphia Evening Bulletin*, August 19, 1919. In his open letter to the editor, Booker T. Washington, Jr., described his experience with housing discrimination in Philadelphia.

[6]Philadelphia Public Ledger, January 26, 1917; Philadelphia Public Ledger, January 31, 1918.

[7]"On Certain Aspects of the Housing Problem in Philadelphia," 3, read by Mr. Crenshaw, mimeograph manuscript, Temple Urban Archive (Philadelphia, PA, 1902).

[8]Bernard Newman, *Housing the City Negro* (Philadelphia, PA: Whittier Centre, 1914), 1–8. Newman served as the Executive Secretary of the Philadelphia Housing Commission. In this report, he offers the result of a study completed on housing conditions among Blacks in Philadelphia. The study was cosponsored by the Whittier Centre, a local civic association. Data were collected by nurses who made site visits to 1,158 homes where 4,891 Blacks lived. Of these homes, 901 lived in the district west of Broad Street and South of Market Street and 257 were in the area east of Broad. The Philadelphia Housing Commission published the full results in 1915.

Frequently, owners of the properties ignored the complaints of occupants and the abatement orders of the Board of Health, and with limited voting rights, blacks had few means to demand improvements.[9]

Despite enjoying a measure of improved social freedom since moving North, many black Philadelphians continued to experience social, economic, and political marginalization. As a group, they were disproportionately poor, residentially segregated, deprived of education, and largely confined to manual labor and domestic work.[10] With limited resources for social welfare relief, the Black community coalesced and when necessary turned inward and formed community institutions such as churches, benevolent clubs, and kinlike networks of support to meet their pressing needs. A 1923 study examining black migrants in Philadelphia found that as many as 90% were churchgoers and 36% belonged to fraternities and sororities.[11] Membership in these organizations offered an opportunity for blacks to meet socially and connect, though perhaps more importantly, it offered a safe place for members to discuss community issues and concerns.

THE "BLACK HEALTH CRISIS," SELF-HELP, AND COMMUNITY HEALTH ACTIVISM

One of the greatest worries among black community residents at the turn of the twentieth century was the high rate of infectious disease in the community. In 1900, tuberculosis (TB) mortality among black Philadelphians was 2 1/2 to 3 times that of native whites.[12] Though the rates of TB declined among all groups in the city during the first decades of the twentieth century,

---

[9]"On Certain Aspects of the Housing Problem in Philadelphia," 3, report as read by Mr. Crenshaw, mimeograph manuscript, Temple Urban Archives (Philadelphia, PA, 1902), URB 46, F2, B13.

[10]William D. Fuller, *Negro Migrant Study* (Philadelphia, PA, Henry Phipps Institute, 1923), 31.

[11]Negro Migration Committee, "Report of the Negro Migration Committee on Housing Conditions of Black Philadelphians," *Pamphlet* (Philadelphia Housing Association, July 9, 1923). The committee on Negro Migration consisted of a host of private and public organizations among them: The Armstron Association, The Children's Bureau, Durham Public School, Federation of Churches, Interracial Committee, Mercy Hospital, Philadelphia Health Council, Octavia Hill Association, and the Philadelphia Housing Association. These associations worked collaboratively to meet the vast social and health needs of Black migrants once they reached the city.

[12]City of Philadelphia, Department of Public Health and Charities, "Annual Report of the Bureau of Health," (1901), 80.

mortality among blacks decreased less rapidly.[13] Much of the excessive illness among black residents was linked to factors such as racism, poverty, and inadequate housing.[14] In addition, local hospitals and private sanitariums often placed restrictions on admitting black patients.[15] Those that did admit blacks, such as Philadelphia General Hospital, often suffered from overcrowding and disrepair.[16] When TB beds were available in less restrictive facilities, some blacks refused to leave the comforts of home due to fear of the treatment they would receive once arriving at the sanatoria and placing themselves under the care of strangers.[17]

Health conditions only seemed to worsen as large waves of new black migrants pressed into the city between 1916 and 1922, taxing the city's already strained municipal infrastructure. The Bureau of Health, the city's most visible arm for sanitation and health, persistently struggled with fiscal constraints and competing objectives related to a variety of public health priorities.[18] Meanwhile, black city residents continued to fall prey to infectious disease leaving many of the health needs of the black community to the efforts of the private sector.[19]

Aware of the public health risk posed by TB and the black community's preference for self-help, the Whittier Center, a local civic association, met in May 1913 to discuss suitable means to thwart the effects of the disease in the community.[20] The Whittier Center was a philanthropic association established in the fall of 1912 and named after the nineteenth-century poet

---

[13]Landis, *A Report of the Tuberculosis Problem and the Negro* Henry Phipps Institute.

[14]Louis T. Wright, "Health Problems of the Negro," *Interracial Review* 8 (January 1935): 6–8.

[15]David McBride, *Integrating the City of Medicine: Blacks in Philadelphia Healthcare, 1910–1965* (Philadelphia, PA: Temple University Press, 1989).

[16]Report of the Committee on Municipal Charities of Philadelphia, *The Report of the Sub-Committee on Tuberculosis* (Philadelphia, PA, 1913), 111–112.

[17]Sadie T. Mossell, *A Study of the Negro Tuberculosis Problem in Philadelphia* (Philadelphia, PA, Henry Phipps Institute, 1923).

[18]By private sector, I refer to private charities and other civic associations such as settlement houses and benevolent societies who provided health and social resources to city residents in the need.

[19]The Bureau of Health TB campaign included broad reform agenda, which included providing funds for sputum collection to diagnose TB, education, and fumigation of homes where TB was found. In a review of Board of Health Annual Reports from 1900 to 1921, no targeted measures were identified toward black city residents despite the notable mortality in this community. See: J. Margo Brooks Carthon, *No Place for the Dying: A Tale of Urban Health Work in Philadelphia's Black Belt, 1900–1930* (Ann Arbor, MI: ProQuest, 2008): 52–68.

[20]Whittier Center Executive Board Meeting Minutes, 1913.

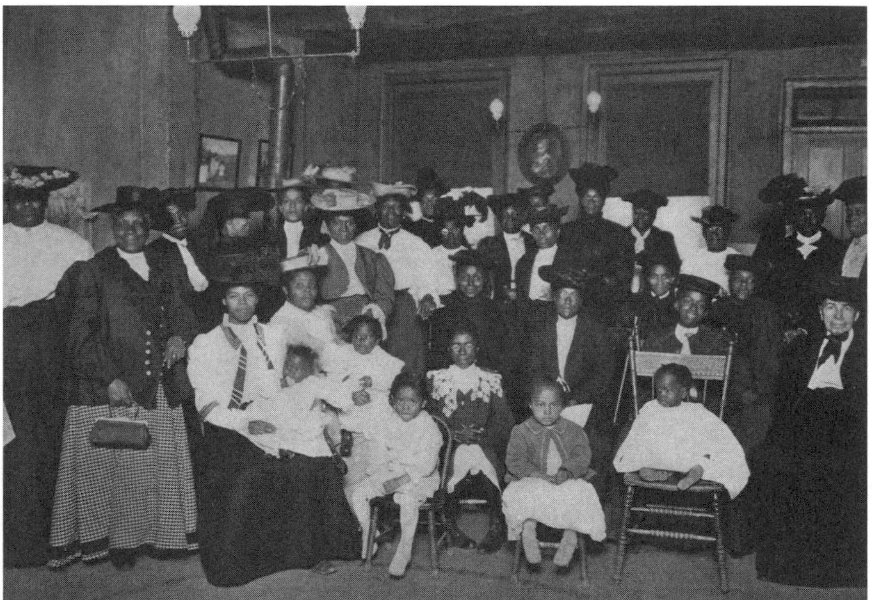

FIGURE 6.1 Co-operative Coal Club. Starr Centre Annual Report (Philadelphia, 1911). *From the Starr Centre Association Collection. Reprinted with the permission of the Barbara Bates Center for the Study of the History of Nursing, School of Nursing, University of Pennsylvania.*

and abolitionist Greenleaf Whittier. The association, comprising black and white civic activists from the local community, formed with a mission to create solutions to the social and health problems plaguing black residents. In its first year, the association focused its efforts toward the members of two black benevolent societies located in South Philadelphia, the Cooperative Coal Club and Rainy Day Society. Both clubs had long historical roots in the black community and together boasted a membership of more than 1,000 individuals.[21]

The first of the two societies, the Coal Club, was formed in 1893 and served as a vehicle for blacks to work collectively to buy coal, then used as a fuel source for cooking and heating homes.[22] Meager weekly wages, however, forced poor and working-class black families to buy it in small amounts, which invariably meant paying higher costs. The Coal Club offered an alternative to these practices by allowing its members to drive down the

---

[21]Whittier Center Annual Report, (Philadelphia, PA, 1914), 4.

[22]Starr Centre Association, Untitled Pamphlet, Barbara Bates Center for the Study of the History of Nursing. Starr Centre Collection, box 9, folder, 105. (Philadelphia, PA, 1907).

price of coal by purchasing it in large amounts together.[23] Club members maintained supportive networks through monthly meetings set aside for social and business purposes.[24] Larger gatherings were often held at local churches, where anywhere between 300 and 400 individuals assembled for health lectures and to discuss club affairs.

Over time, discussions about illness at Coal Club meetings led members to form the Rainy Day Society in 1905. Similar to many other sick benefit societies operating in cities across the country, the Rainy Day Society served as a safety net to its members by providing financial assistance in the event of unexpected illness. Individuals gained membership in the Society through annual dues, which they were able to withdraw in times of illness, or the total savings could be pulled at the beginning of each year for other purchases. Paid staff made weekly personal visits to the home of each member and collected contributions.[25] By 1913, both clubs were well-recognized entities within the black community, and though the Whittier Center itself was a new association, many of its board members had long-standing relationships with black club members. These relationships and the pervasive threat of TB prompted Whittier Center leaders to discuss the merits of hiring a black nurse to investigate for possible cases of TB among members of the black community.[26]

In a meeting of the executive committee on May 14, 1913, TB expert and Whittier Center president, Henry Landis voiced the advantages of this proposition, saying, "to really get behind the scenes" of health conditions in black homes, it would require a person of the same race.[27] This nurse would visit black families and according to Landis, more easily gain their confidence and dispel any fears or superstitions regarding illness that might prevent them from seeking care. Once hired, her duties would be that of a visiting nurse, sanitary inspector, and social worker. She was expected to not only work in the community but also to live in the district and establish a "neighborhood house," where she would serve as a liaison between community members and the association's health objectives. The Whittier Center's proposal to hire a black nurse was at the time regarded as quite a novel experiment. Up to this point, there is little evidence to suggest that black clinicians held prominent positions

---

23Starr Centre Association, *Board of Directors Meeting Minutes* (Philadelphia, PA, July 13, 1911).
24Starr Center Association, *Board of Directors Meeting Minutes* (July 13), 1911.
25Starr Centre Association Annual Report (Philadelphia, PA, 1911), 10; Susan P. Wharton, Negro Branch of the Starr Centre (1909): 16.
26Whittier Center Executive Board Meeting Minutes (1913).
27Whittier Centere Annual Report (Philadelphia, PA, 1915), 3.

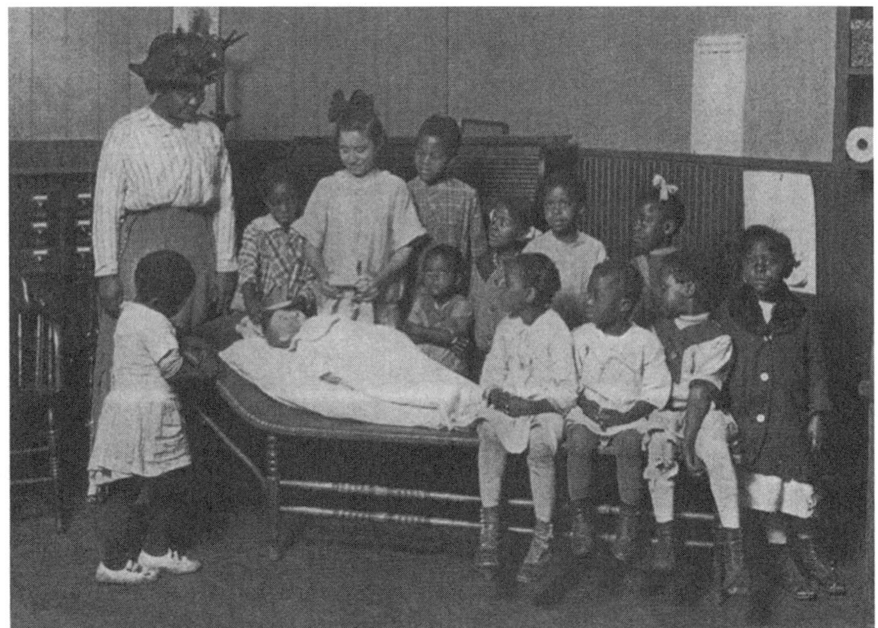

FIGURE 6.2 Elizabeth Tyler. Whittier Center Annual Report (Philadelphia, PA, 1915). *Reprinted with permission from the Temple University Libraries Urban Archives.*

in the anti-TB campaign in Philadelphia.[28] At this meeting, however, the progressive members of the Whittier Center board of director took a step away from tradition and on that day agreed to provide the salary of 65 dollars per month to hire its first black nurse—Elizabeth Tyler.

RACE, PLACE, AND NURSING

Tyler began her new position on February 1, 1914, providing services to the Phipps Institute (established in 1903 as the nation's first endowed center for research and clinical campaigns to prevent and eradicate TB).[29] As a member

---

[28]Sadie T. Mossell, *A Study of The Negro Tuberculosis Problem in Philadelphia* (Philadelphia, PA: Henry Phipps Institute, 1923); Landis, *A Report of the Tuberculosis Problem and the Negro*.

[29]For more on Phipps, see Barbara Bates, *Bargaining for Life. A Social History of Tuberculosis, 1876–1939* (Philadelphia, PA: University of Pennsyvania Press, 1992); David McBride, "The Henry Phipps Institute, 1903–1937: Pioneering Tuberculosis Work with an Urban Minority," *Bulletin of Medicine*, (1987) vol. 61, no. 1, pp. 78-97.

of the Phipps Institute staff, Tyler's job included finding black residents suspected of TB, then referring them to the Phipps clinic for treatment. Hers was a daunting task; "how to do this," mused Tyler prior to beginning her work, "was a serious question."[30] Tyler knew well that prior to her arrival, few blacks sought care for TB despite the Phipps clinic's central location in the heart of the city's historical black district.

Tyler's education and past professional experience had prepared her well for her new task. As a graduate of Freedman's Hospital Training School in Washington, DC, she was the recipient of a first-class education. After graduation, she worked as a private duty nurse in Northampton, Massachusetts, and then as the resident nurse and instructor of physiology and hygiene at A & M College in Normal, Alabama. In 1906, she accepted a position as the first black visiting nurse of the Henry Street Settlement in New York City.[31] During her time as a public health nurse in New York, she worked among poor black and immigrant families with health concerns similar to those that she would face once arriving to Philadelphia.

Tyler's first year in Philadelphia was spent providing home care to 327 families that were intimately affiliated with the Whittier Center. The number of persons in these families totaled well over 1,000 and included a large number of Coal Club and Rainy Day Society members.[32] Of those members visited, 12% were suspected of having TB and were subsequently referred to the hospital or clinic for treatment. Once receiving fair treatment at the TB clinic, patients then referred friends and family to the clinic for similar care. Of this response, Tyler noted, "It is gratifying to know that the number of colored people attending the Phipps Institute has been so greatly increased as a direct result of these house-to house investigations."[33] In the first year of her work in Philadelphia, the number of black patients who visited the clinic was 12 times more than those who had visited during the first 11 years of the Institute's history. So effective were these efforts that within 6 months of her hire, another black nurse, Cora Johnson, was added to the Phipps Institute staff. Later that same year, a black physician, Henry Minton, joined to oversee the care of black patients at the dispensary, their salaries paid by the Philadelphia Committee of the Pennsylvania Society for the Study of Tuberculosis and the Pennsylvania State Department of Health.[34]

---

[30]Whittier Center Annual Report (Philadelphia, PA, 1914), 4.

[31]Marie O. Pitts Mosely, "Satisfied to Carry the Bag: Three Black Community Health Nurses Contributions to Health Reform, 1900–1937," *Nursing History Review* 4 (1996): 65–82.

[32]Whittier Center Annual Report (Philadelphia, PA, 1914), 6.

[33]Whittier Center Annual Report (Philadelphia, PA, 1914), quote found on p. 7.

[34]Whittier Center Annual Report (Philadelphia, PA, 1915), 6.

Instrumental to Tyler's success was her ability to extend her nursing care to areas beyond the boundaries of health. During her home visits, Tyler first built a strong rapport with neighborhood families and then inquired about the health conditions of their families and their housing and economic concerns. In her first year, Tyler found that nearly 62% of the families visited required medical or social services. For Tyler, this meant offering advice, making referrals to other civic agencies, or recommending treatment at the Phipps Institute. As a result, Tyler was recognized as an important community resource—working closely with families, civic leaders, and other health professionals. In January 1914, Tyler along with Drs. Minton and Landis launched the Committee on Health and Sanitation for the purpose of planning and executing health activities for the members of the clubs. The committee's efforts included holding health lectures in local churches. Four such lectures were held during the winter of 1914 with nearly 1,500 people in attendance.[35]

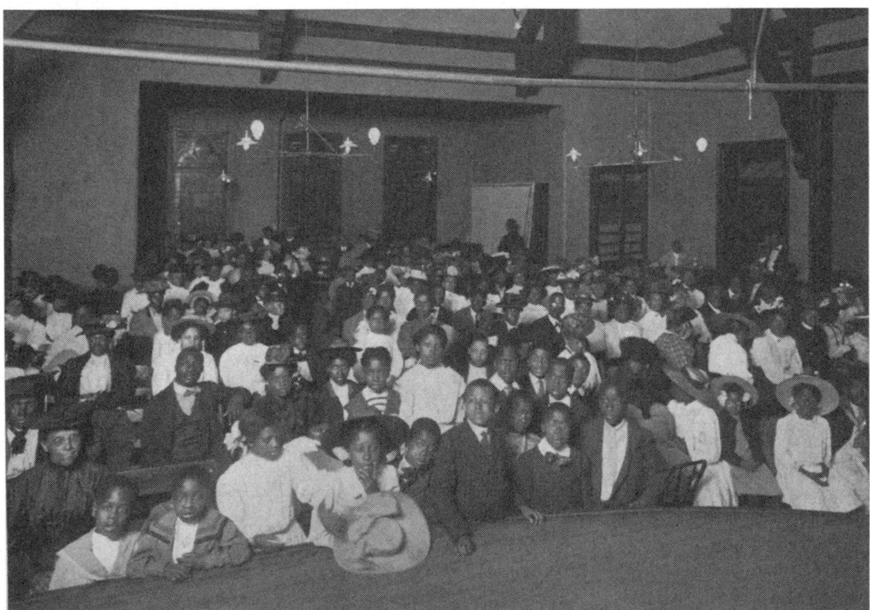

FIGURE 6.3 Coal Club Ready for the Lesson. Starr Centre Annual Report (Philadelphia, 1906). *Starr Centre Association Collection. Reprinted with permission of the Barbara Bates Center for the Study of the History of Nursing, School of Nursing, University of Pennsylvania.*

---

[35]Whittier Center Annual Report (Philadelphia, PA, 1916), 6.

Tyler was also a health educator and during her first year in Philadelphia helped to organize three "Little Mother Clubs" in the neighborhood. As members of the clubs, girls received lessons on hygiene, breastfeeding, and childcare, which were used as a means to reduce infant mortality in the city. In addition to these activities, Tyler helped to organize a club composed of women in the immediate neighborhood who desired to address community issues.[36] This club along with the other activities of the Whittier Center solidified Tyler's base and allowed her to introduce health promotion initiatives in concert with other community building efforts. Over the decade following her hire, the Whittier Center's involvement with community health grew to include the establishment of several health centers, including a prenatal clinic, well-baby clinics, and home supervision. By 1927, the staff of black clinicians, then known as the Negro Health Bureau, grew from 1 nurse to 10 and from 1 physician to 12.[37]

Despite Tyler's overall successes in increasing health awareness, it would be misleading to present her only in light of her accomplishments, as she often felt that she was "just scratching the surface" and that there were "gaps and leaks in the system which caused failure in too many cases."[38] In several instances, sick individuals refused to leave their unhygienic surroundings; others failed to improve under any circumstances. In 1916 during a routine investigation, Tyler came across a man bedridden with a "bad cold." After much coercion, the man sought treatment at the Phipps Institute and was diagnosed with TB, though he refused inpatient treatment until the woman with whom he was lodging could no longer provide him food. When he was finally admitted to Philadelphia General Hospital, he died after only 3 weeks of care. Despite having the home fumigated, the woman of the house soon became ill with TB; she was likely infected by the lodger. In cases such as these, Tyler believed that there was no protection for noninfected members of the household, "Had the man been discovered earlier, the woman might be in good health today."[39]

---

[36]Whittier Center Annual Report, (Philadelphia, PA, 1914), 4–5.

[37]Henry R. M. Landis, *The Work of the Whittier Centre* (Philadelphia, PA, Philadelphia Housing Association, 1927), 5. Landis notes that the additional Black clinical staff was made possible by funding through the Philadelphia Health Council. The Whittier Center Annual Report (Philadelphia, PA, 1924), 3; 14. The 1924 annual report offers a brief description of the Negro Health Bureau, which served as a branch of the Whittier Center, under the direction of Dr. H. M. Minton. The Bureau was responsible for oversight for several clinics primarily attended by Blacks. They included Health Center no. 1 at the Henry Phipps Institute, Health Clinic no. 2 at Jefferson Hospital, and Health Clinic no. 3 at Twentieth and Ridge Avenue. Health Center no. 3 was added in March 1923 due to the large overflow of patients in the first two clinics.

[38]Whittier Center Annual Report (Philadelphia, PA, 1916), 6.

[39]Whittier Center Annual Report (Philadelphia, PA, 1916), 6.

Tyler points to early detection as the surest way to prevent further spread of illness. This case, however, illustrates something else, perhaps more profound. As a visiting home nurse, Tyler surely recognized that understanding an individual's response to illness starts first with assessing their contextual reality. The woman in this case relied on this boarder as a means to supplement her income, never realizing perhaps that there were risks involved—threats to her own well-being. For many blacks, the practice of taking in boarders opened a de facto contractual relationship, one where economics and personal space overlapped.This exchange of living space for money, however, left both parties vulnerable to the health practices, or *nonpractices*, of one another. Pressing economic needs often forced blacks to think first of their livelihoods—these choices, however, often cost them their lives.[40]

Despite experiencing her share of setbacks, Tyler's work with the Whittier Center and Phipps Institute represents an extremely successful and compelling illustration of urban health work conducted during the early twentieth century. As predicted by Whittier Center board members, the addition of black clinicians was an added value to the association's campaign against TB. As a member of the black community, Tyler was able to leverage her racial identity to establish trust and increase buy-in from community residents to promote important, life-saving health initiatives. She did this, however, while recognizing the value of community networks and institutions operating in the community prior to her arrival and partnering with community members who were active participants in health initiatives during this period.[41] After identifying these resources, Tyler combined community organizing with relationship building and health advocacy with providing social and material

---

[40]Whittier Center Annual Report (Philadelphia, PA, 1919), 6.

[41]Elizabeth Tyler's career as a public health nurse did not end in Philadelphia. In 1921, she left the Henry Phipps Institute to take a position in Delaware for the State Health and Welfare Commission. Later she held positions in Newark and Essex County, New Jersey, for the N.J. Tuberculosis League and the Essex County Tuberculosis League, respectively. In each position, Tyler maintained her community outreach efforts for the purposes of education and disease prevention. In the current examination of Tyler's pubic health activities, I attempt to layer Tyler's nursing work alongside those of civically active community residents and thereby recontextualize her health promotion success within the larger scope of community-building initiatives already perculating in local Black communities. For a broader treatment of Tyler's career as a public health nurse, see Marie O. Pitts Mosely, "Satisfied to Carry the Bag: Three Black Community Health Nurses; Contributions to Health Care Reform, 1900–1937," in *Nurses Across Time and Place*, ed. Patricia D'Antonio and Ellen D. Baer (Springer Publishing, New York, 2007), 73–74.

support. These *collective* measures helped to establish a collaborative model of community health, which helped to foster relevant program planning for the neighborhood under her care.

CONCLUSION

This chapter draws on the long history of nurses who for more than a century have provided care in the neighborhoods and homes of the most vulnerable people in America. Much of their success stemmed from their ability to establish relationships, build trust, and form partnerships with neighborhood residents. Some of the more successful examples of community nursing throughout the last century incorporated a collaborative model, which included residents of the community in the planning and implementation of health initiatives. Hence, while this chapter focuses on *nursing* care measures, its purpose is not to highlight *a specific* nursing intervention, which may be transported through time. Instead, it offers a set of principles evident nearly a century ago, which may be used to influence "best practices" for nurses providing care to diverse patients in community settings today. It also serves as a reminder that nursing interventions are inextricably connected to the context where they take place—and that the inhabitants, values, and cultural attributes of communities must be taken into account for health changes to occur.

ACKNOWLEDGMENTS

This research was supported by the Agency for Healthcare Research and Quality (Grant F-31 HS01029-02), National Institutes of Health, and National Institute of Nursing Research (Grants R01-NR04513 and T32-NR0714). Portions of this manuscript have been published previously in the *Nursing History Review*.

CHAPTER 7

Filling the Gaps in Community Care: Parish Nurses Working Out of Congregations

Lisa M. Zerull

INTRODUCTION

For more than a century, national concern for public welfare and how best to address unmet healthcare needs have challenged political, social, and religious support structures. While recent legislature addresses the question of health insurance coverage for the majority, it does not fully address access to preventative care. Other creative strategies are needed to fill the gaps in care, especially in the community setting, where services are frequently lacking. While hospitals provide illness care and public agencies offer limited healthcare resources, there exists opportunity for community organizations to take more active roles in health promotion. For example, churches have historically reached out to the community to help those in need when no other resources were available.

Throughout history, the church has been an integral part of the health, healing, and social well-being of a community.[1] Nurses have a long history of association with churches, namely the Catholic sisters and Protestant deaconesses who promoted health and cared for the sick and the poor for

[1]Steve Wilhide, "Commentary," in *Rural Roads: A Quarterly Magazine*, no. 2 (National Rural Health Association, June 2004), 2.

centuries.[2] In particular, the deaconess nurses associated with the Baltimore Lutheran Deaconess Motherhouse beginning in 1895 were known for their parish work. Parish deaconesses were trained as nurses and worked out of an assigned church or parish to provide a unique combination of nursing, spiritual, and social care for the city's urban poor. In this chapter, the Lutheran antecedents to contemporary faith-based nursing initiatives are examined taking into consideration the social, cultural, economic, and healthcare delivery context of the period. Examining how Lutheran deaconesses worked out of parishes and provided nursing care in the community may identify creative initiatives adaptable to twenty-first-century nursing.

THE SETTING OF BALTIMORE IN THE 1890S

On October 9, 1895, with six women formally trained as nurses, the doors of the Baltimore Lutheran Deaconess Motherhouse and Training School opened in a suburban row house located at 907 North Fulton Avenue to serve the surrounding community.[3] Fully supported by the regional Lutheran churches, the geographic selection of Baltimore for a deaconess motherhouse was ideal. Second only to New York City in size in the 1890s, Baltimore's population of 450,000 was culturally diverse, made up of immigrants from Germany, Poland, Italy, and Russia. First- and second-generation German Americans, many of whom were Lutherans, comprised almost a quarter of Baltimore's total population. In addition, a large number of blacks migrated from the rural South to Baltimore. Most were poor and

---

[2]Quote by John Mason Neale in Anne Doyle "Nursing by Religious Orders in the United States: Part IV—Lutheran Deaconesses, 1849–1928," *American Journal of Nursing* 29 (1929), 1204. See also, Phyllis Ann Solari-Twadell and Karen Egenes, "A Historical Perspective of Parish Nursing: Rules for the Sisters of the Parishes," in *Parish Nursing: Development, Education, and Administration* (St. Louis, MO: Elsevier Mosby, 2006), 11–16. See also Theodor Fliedner, *Some Account of the Deaconess-Work in the Christian Church* (Kaiserswerth, Germany: Sam Lucas, 1870), 26. Roman Catholic sisters beginning in 1633 with Vincent de Paul in Paris, France, and Protestant deaconesses beginning at Kaiserswerth, Germany, in 1836 with Theodor Fliedner were formally trained as nurses and provided wholistic care to the poor and the sick.

[3]Lucy Eyster, *Diary #1 February 14–Dec 23, 1893*, Evangelical Lutheran Church in America Archives (hereafter cited as ELCAA), ELCA 127/6/1, Deceased Personnel Files, box 11, folder 1.

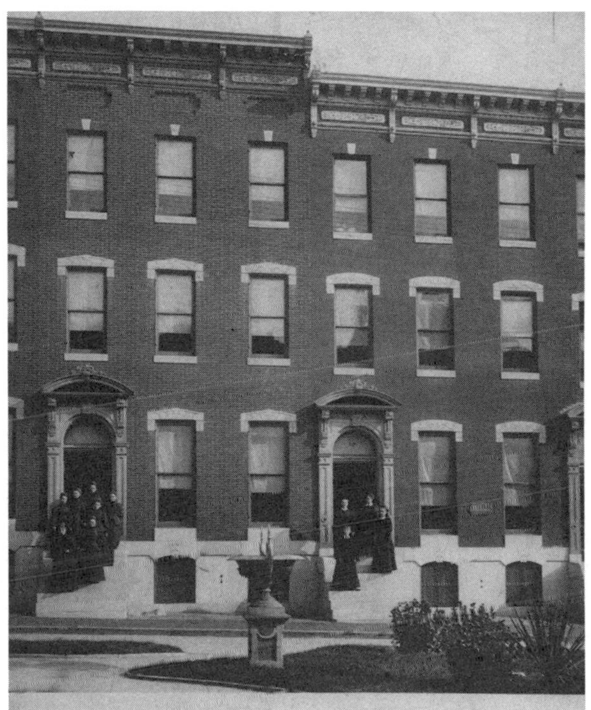

FIGURE 7.1 Baltimore Lutheran Deaconess Motherhouse, ca. 1896. *Reprinted with permission of The Evangelical Lutheran Church in America Archives (Elk Grove Village, IL).*

possessed few marketable job skills for an urban setting. All were vying to earn a living in jobs associated with industry, transportation, and domestic service.

These men, women, and children settling in to Baltimore's overcrowded row houses struggled to survive the realities of existence. Abject poverty, crime, inadequate sanitation, and infectious diseases such as tuberculosis and typhoid were the norm among the poor. Increasing tensions with race relations and widening disparities between social classes became obvious. In response, the middle and upper classes mobilized resources and engaged in community support as members of charitable organizations such as the Red Cross, Salvation Army, and Settlement Houses. Joining in their efforts were Protestants, Catholics, and Jews who provided religious and social support as well as physical care to persons in need.

Overall, the Baltimoreans possessed a strong sense of civic idealism, particularly the middle and upper classes intent upon municipal betterment, progressivism, and bringing about much-needed political, economic, and social reforms.[4] With the overwhelming needs of the poor, there was growing social acceptance of women moving beyond the confines of home and family to explore new opportunities for education and expanding roles in the public sphere. This was true for the women who became Lutheran deaconesses, and it was in this social context that the women became a nursing presence in the Baltimore community.

THE LUTHERAN DEACONESS NURSE

The Baltimore Deaconess Motherhouse was organized and directed by the larger church body of the Lutheran General Synod. Promoting the female deaconess role was a new departure for its membership given its history of support to male-dominated ministries. With the patriarchal mindsets of the time period, the paradigm shift of supporting acceptable female roles outside the home challenged the thinking of many. Lutherans intentionally promoted the deaconess role as an office of the church.[5] This delineation elevated the status of women's work in the church and encouraged social acceptance. Moreover, while nineteenth-century deaconesses were embraced by individual Protestant churches in specific locations, no other organized church body in American Lutheranism made provision for this kind of recognition or control of the female diaconate role.[6] Indeed, as stated by one clergy in support of the new Baltimore Motherhouse, the deaconess role proposed was organized "in a Church, *by* a Church, *of* a Church, and [created] *for* the Church."[7]

---

[4]Samuel Zenas Ammen, "History of Baltimore: 1875–1895," in *Baltimore: Its History and Its People*, ed. Clayton Colman Hall (New York: Lewis Historical Publishing, 1912), 243.
[5]Julie Mergner, *The Deaconess and Her Work*, trans. Mrs. Adolph Spaeth (Philadelphia, PA: General Council Publishing House, 1915), 9. See also, The Board of Deaconess Work, *Minutes* (Baltimore, MD: United Lutheran Church in America, n.d.—ca. 1918), ELCAA, ULCA BOARD History, Orders of Service, Anniversaries, The Board of Deaconess Work, n.d., 1901, 1903, 1905, 1907, 1909, Microform, 3. The German deaconess model provided the foundation of training and service for seven Lutheran motherhouses established in America before 1900. The first American Lutheran motherhouse was organized in 1884 in Philadelphia. Six additional Lutheran motherhouses were established before 1900 in Brooklyn, New York (1885); Omaha, Nebraska (1887), Minneapolis, Minnesota (1889); Milwaukee, Wisconsin (1893); Baltimore, Maryland (1895); and Chicago, Illinois (1897)—wherever large numbers of German and Scandinavian Lutheran immigrants settled in America
[6]The Board of Deaconess Work, *Minutes*, Microform, 3. See also, Frederick Sheely Weiser, "The Origins of Lutheran Deaconesses in America," *Lutheran Quarterly* 13 (1999): 430.
[7]Albert H. Studebaker, "Sermon Address 1901," *LDM & Training School, Baltimore, MD Motherhouse Subject Files 1886–1962*, ELCAA, ULCA 61/5/3, Subject Files 1886–1962, box 7, folder 1, 2.

Borrowing from the German Lutheran traditions of the nineteenth century, the deaconess role combined nursing with the Lutheran theology of "living your faith in active service to another."[8] A Kaiserswerth, Germany, publication from 1883 defined a deaconess as:

> A Protestant Christian woman trained in the Apostolic sense, for the purpose of ministering to the sick, the poor, children, prisoners, released criminals, and the like . . . [the role] endeavors to enlist in the services of the Church the vast fund of womanly love and power, which too often lies dormant, but only requires objects of compassion to quicken into activity . . . [it] extends to the needy of all religions, without any distinction.[9]

This definition recognizes the earliest biblical reference to a female diaconate role (A.D. 60) when St. Paul sent deaconess Phoebe to care for the people

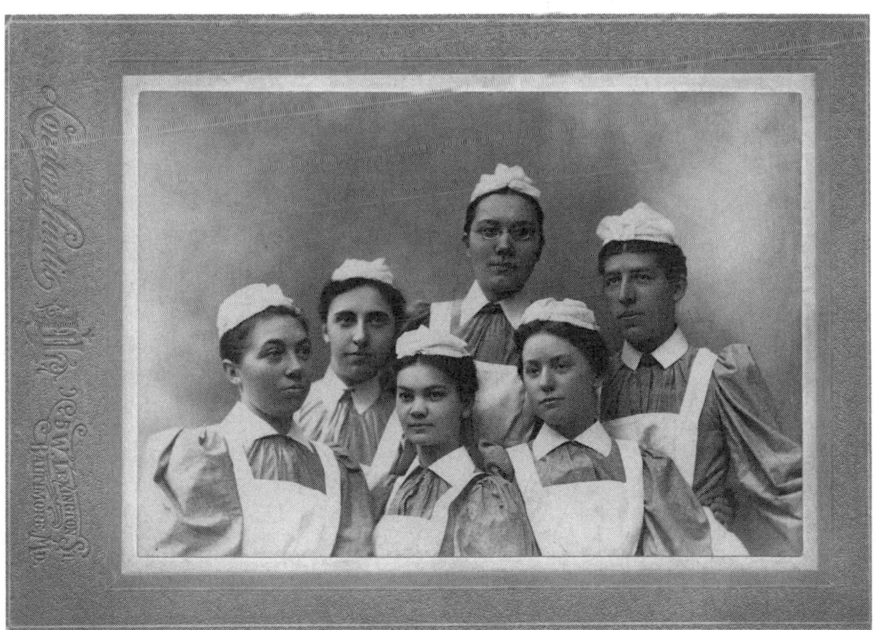

FIGURE 7.2 Six Baltimore Lutheran deaconesses, ca. 1895. *Reprinted with permission of The Evangelical Lutheran Church in America Archives (Elk Grove Village, IL).*

---

[8]Martin Luther, "The Works of Martin Luther," (Philadelphia edition, 1915–1943 in Vol. 6), quoted in Frederick S. Weiser, *Love's Response* (The Board of Publication of the United Lutheran Church in America: Philadelphia), 25.

[9]Julius Disselhoff, *Kaiserswerth: The Deaconess Institution of Rhenish Westphalia, Its Origin and Fields of Labour*, trans. A.N. (London, UK: Hatchards, Piccadilly, 1883), 7.

of Cenchreae.[10] Phoebe was a woman well regarded because of her faith, education, wealth, and position.[11] Following a Christian example, Phoebe, and the countless numbers of widows and unmarried woman who succeeded her, served the church through compassionate acts of mercy. These early church initiatives provided care to the poor and the sick when no other care was available beyond family members or acquaintances.

Just as deaconess Phoebe was carefully selected for her work of service in Apostolic times, so, too, were the women of the Baltimore Motherhouse chosen to take the deaconess training. The motherhouse's *Handbook of the Deaconess Work* (1895) called for "single women and childless widows from 20 to 40 years old, of blameless reputation, in good health, with capacity for receiving instructions, and a right spirit" to make application.[12] Two of the six original women who entered the Baltimore Motherhouse were pursuing academic degrees in Chicago at the time of their selection. Almost all were from rural communities and possessed a satisfactory level of education. Overall, the women were spiritually and emotionally mature, possessing the potential to carry out the combined professional and domestic responsibilities expected of the deaconess in the communal living environment of the motherhouse, and in the provision of nursing care.

The deaconess training was comprehensive and combined medicine, science, religion, and nursing. The period of instruction took a minimum of 2 years with some variation in length according to a woman's capabilities, knowledge, and experience.[13] Four broad areas of deaconess study included religious and theoretical education along with general studies focused on writing and mathematics in the classroom and practical experience in caring for patients. Physicians and deaconesses taught the medical, theoretical, and practical nursing courses, while the Lutheran clergy provided the religious and spiritual instruction that encompassed church and deaconess history, theology, and bible study.[14] In addition, self-care was encouraged through daily exercise, fellowship with other deaconesses, and outdoor activities. Also

---

[10]Romans 16:1–2 (New International Version). "I commend to you our sister Phoebe, a servant of the church in Cenchrea. I ask you to receive her in the Lord in a way worthy of the saints and to give her any help she may need from you, for she has been a great help to many people, including me."

[11]Fliedner, *Some Account of the Deaconess-Work*, 3–4.

[12]Board of Deaconess Work, *Hand-book of the Deaconess Board of the General Synod in the United States* (Philadelphia, PA: Lutheran Publication Society Print, 1895), ELCAA, ULCA 61/8/1, Handbook/ Catalogue, Lutheran Deaconess Motherhouse and Training School, 1895, 1903–1947, box 2, folder 2, 9–10.

[13]Disselhoff, *Kaiserswerth*, 8. See also, Mergner, *The Deaconess and Her Work*, 95–96.

[14]Board of Deaconess Work, *Hand-book*, 22–23.

included as important components of training were the domestic responsibilities of cleaning, laundering, sewing, and food preparation.[15] Overall, the deaconess training was rigorous and intended to teach women to properly care for the body and soul of those they served.[16]

In addition to providing a place of protection and refuge in sickness or old age, the motherhouse was where the deaconesses combined everyday living with academics, worship, and service.[17] The motherhouse provided shelter and food, along with the deaconess uniform or garb complete with the signature Baltimore cross pin, and all expenses associated with education and the carrying out the deaconess work. The value of teamwork and Christian communal living was recognized and provided spiritual sustenance to the

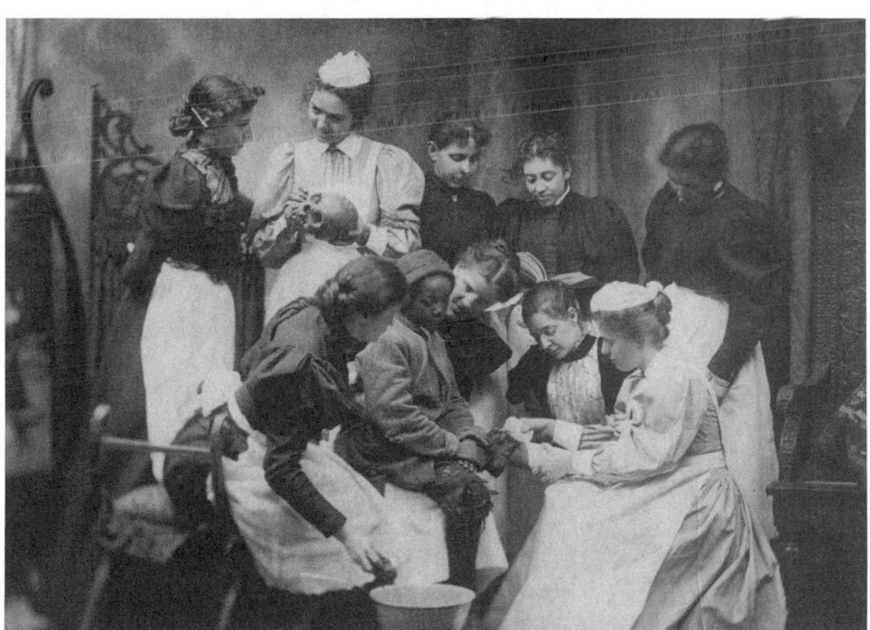

FIGURE 7.3 Deaconess classroom, ca. 1898. *Reprinted with permission of The Evangelical Lutheran Church in America Archives (Elk Grove Village, IL)*

---

[15]Jennie Christ, *Daybook No. 1: January 1894–April 1894*, ELCAA, ELCA 127/6/1, Deceased Personnel Files, 1884–2003, box 8, folder 7, quote from January 2, 1894.

[16]Fliedner, *Some Account of the Deaconess-Work*, 11–15. See also, Abdel Ross Wentz, *Fliedner the Faithful* (Philadelphia, PA: The Board of Publication of the United Lutheran Church in America, 1936), 48.

[17]Board of Deaconess Work, *Hand-book*, 17.

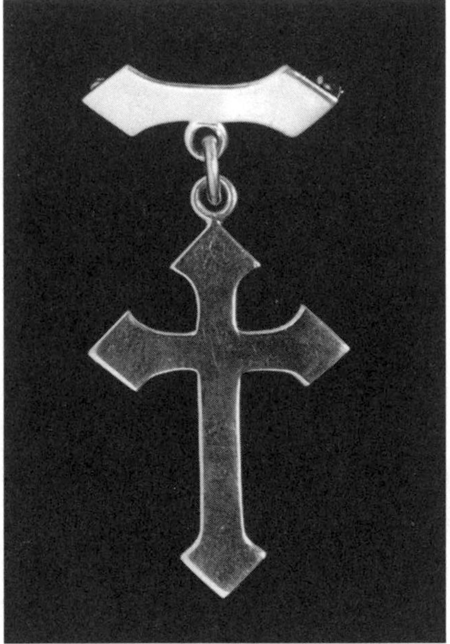

FIGURE 7.4 Baltimore Motherhouse cross worn as a pin by consecrated deaconesses, ca. 1898. *Reprinted with permission of The Evangelical Lutheran Church in America Archives (Elk Grove Village, IL).*

many women brought together by common purpose and calling.[18] Present in every motherhouse, including Baltimore, was a formal chapel or worship space for the deaconesses to participate in daily rituals of faith, including worship, prayer, and meditation. Intentional spiritual nurturing of the deaconesses proved to sustain them in their work over time.[19]

BALTIMORE DEACONESS SERVICE TO THE COMMUNITY

In beginning of the deaconess work in Baltimore, the motherhouse leadership realized the immediate need of obtaining income while also gaining public recognition of the deaconess work. Thus, for the first year of operations,

---

[18]Ibid., 35–36.

[19]Jennie Christ, *Daybook No. 2: July 1895–September 1896*, ELCAA, ELCA 127/6/1 Deceased Personnel Files, box 8, folder 8.

deaconesses were assigned to nurse persons in their homes diagnosed with cancer, typhoid, tuberculosis, and dysentery.[20] As noted by deaconess Jennie Christ (pronounced krĭst) in her diary entry dated Sunday, November 3, 1895:

> A nurse was needed way out on Cross street. A case of typhoid. I volunteered to go. When I came I found my patient quite sick and yet not so dangerous as most cases of this kind are. The family is very grateful for all we do and yet in a work like ours we must expect to work very often when we received no encouragement only trust to God for the future fruits.[21]

Christ's diary entry reflects the confidence of a trained deaconess in providing the necessary nursing care to a patient ill with an infectious disease. Aware of the real possibility that she may contract the disease, Christ's faith and motivation to serve others regardless of reward replaced any fear for her own well-being. Motherhouse records identified only minor illnesses of the deaconesses. None of the original six Baltimore women succumbed to an infectious disease.[22]

In addition to private nursing, the motherhouse and its deaconesses offered educational outreach to the Baltimore community. The women taught Sunday School at multiple Lutheran churches and provided three youth education programs to the surrounding community out of the motherhouse that included a weekday kindergarten, an industrial school, and a night school for those they called "colored" children.[23] The education programs reflected the diversity of the families living in the neighborhoods surrounding the motherhouse and the commitment to reach out to area Lutherans and to others in need of resources, ministry, and education.

By promoting the deaconess service at the motherhouse, in churches, and to community organizations, word about the good work of the Baltimore deaconesses soon spread. By 1896, the motherhouse doubled the available space by expanding to the adjacent row house to accommodate six additional women.[24] The steady income from private nursing and donations provided sufficient financial resources for the motherhouse to assign trained deaconesses as parish workers in Lutheran congregations.

---

[20]Augusta Shaffer, *Daily Record of Events Occurring in the Lutheran Deaconess Motherhouse*, ELCAA, ULCA 61/5/3, box 1, folder 10.
[21]Christ, *Daybook No. 2*.
[22]Baltimore Deaconess Motherhouse, *Register of Deaconesses 1892–1970*, vol. 1, ELCAA, ULCA 61/5/4, Deaconess Notebooks and Lists 1892–1972, box 1, folder 1.
[23]Lina Schueler, *Reminiscence*, ELCAA, ULCA 61/1/1 BMD Histories, Handwritten, Typewritten Reminiscences by Deaconesses, ND-1934, box 1, folder 4, 1–2.
[24]Shaffer, *Daily Record of Events*, 5.

PARISH DEACONESSES

The Baltimore Motherhouse would become well known for the training of women as parish deaconesses. As the population of Baltimore increased, so did the numbers of church members in Lutheran congregations. While trying to meet the needs of growing congregations, clergy were challenged to minister to others in the community beyond its membership. In seeking additional support for its ministry, the congregation had the option of hiring either an assistant pastor or a parish deaconess. Often the deciding factor to request a parish deaconess was that churches did not need additional preaching and performing of ministerial acts. Rather, they sought a trained deaconess to bridge the gap between the pastor's work and meeting the physical and social needs of the congregation and surrounding community.[25] The parish deaconess brought new and varied skills that complemented the ministry of the male clergy.

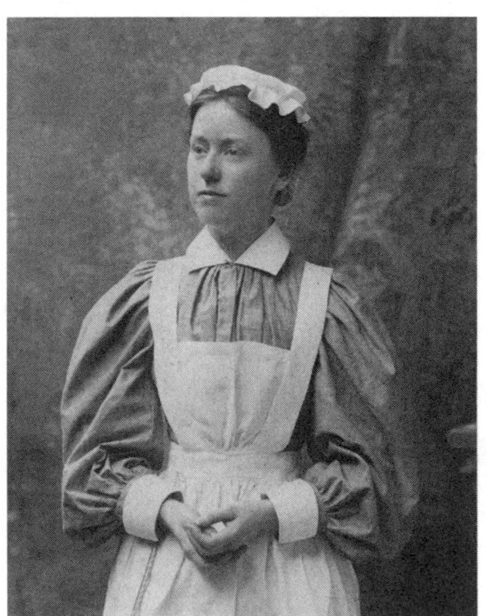

FIGURE 7.5 Sister Jennie Christ in nursing garb, ca. 1896. *Reprinted with permission of The Evangelical Lutheran Church in America Archives (Elk Grove Village, IL).*

---

[25]Mergner, *The Deaconess and Her Work,* 140.

The responsibilities of the parish deaconess varied and were broad in scope. After a woman completed the required 2 years of classroom studies and nurse training, she began additional studies that focused on teaching and parish work.[26] An early text used for deaconess training purposes identified that "there was scarcely any talent or any accomplishment that a woman has ever cultivated that cannot be made useful by the right kind of *parish sister.*"[27] Once assigned to a congregation, the parish deaconess received direction from the pastor and church council while continuing to maintain ties with the motherhouse. The deaconess's duties varied depending upon the needs of the congregation and the priorities of its leadership. In this excerpt taken from a two-page flyer written by a Baltimore clergy, the duties of a deaconess assigned to parish work are described:

> This spiritual ministry includes conferences on spiritual experiences, reading of the Scriptures and prayer with the sick and the shut-ins. It also involves the looking up of Sunday School scholars, the contacting of the homes of those who have recently taken up their abode in the community, or just a purely social call . . . ministering such pastoral care as she is fitted to minister.[28]

Evidence of value of the nursing role was found in this quote by a Baltimore clergy: "Her visits had not been perfunctory, but thoroughly intelligent and effective. Her report, though modest and deprecatory of self, showed that her coming was a real God-send to more than one of the households visited."[29] In addition to home visits, parish deaconesses carried out their work in multiple settings throughout the community, including the church, public places, hospitals, and institutions of care. The majority of referrals were received from the clergy who directed her to the cases of most pressing need. Other referrals came from parishioner families and from church-based groups, such as the King's Daughters or Ladies Sewing Circle.[30]

Parish deaconess care was based upon the needs of those she visited. During a home visit on April 25, 1896, deaconess Lucy Eyster's nursing note describes her nursing care that combined the domestic task of cleaning her

---

[26]Ruth Rasche, *The Deaconess Heritage: One Hundred Years of Caring, Healing and Teaching* (St. Louis, MO: The Deaconess Foundation, 1994), 280.
[27]Mergner, *The Deaconess and Her Work,* 142.
[28]Samuel T. Nicholas, *The Pastor and the Deaconess* (Baltimore, MD: Lutheran Deaconess Motherhouse and Training School, ca. 1900, Wentz Library of the Lutheran Seminary at Gettysburg [hereafter cited as WLLTSG]), series 9, 2.
[29]William S. Freas, *The Parish Deaconess,* WLLTSG, series 9, box 2, 4–5.
[30]Shaffer, *Daily Record of Events*, 5.

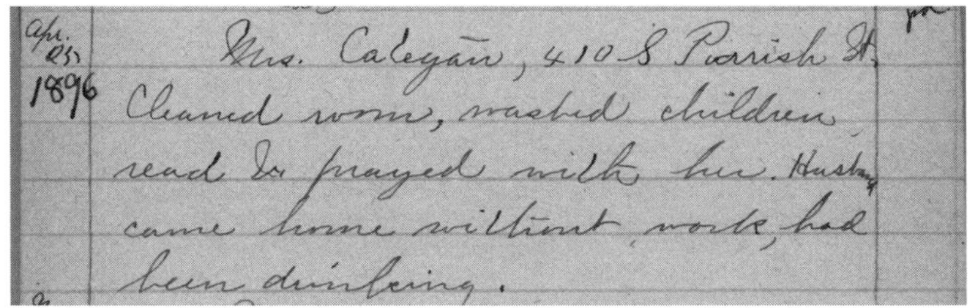
Apr. 25, 1896 Mrs. Calegan, 410 S Parrish St.
Cleaned room, washed children
read & prayed with her. Husb.
came home without work, had
been drinking.

FIGURE 7.6 Nursing note of Sister Lucy Eyster dated April 25, 1896. *Reprinted with permission of The Evangelical Lutheran Church in America Archives (Elk Grove Village, IL).*

patient's room with spiritual care offered in the form of a prayer. Eyster also identifies the social concerns of unemployment and alcoholism frequently found in the homes of the poor.[31] Similarly, deaconess Jennie Christ wrote about the realities of Baltimore's poor during a visit with a man bed-bound with rheumatism. "When I entered the home I found a warm fire (*industry succeeds*) and I did not stop long to speak with wife and daughter but went directly to the room where my patient lay. After hearing how he felt I read to him and we had a prayer."[32] With almost every deaconess visit, some form of spiritual care was documented such as prayer, the reading of scripture, singing hymns, or offering a supportive presence.[33] The deaconess served as the human link connecting faith to health for parishioners in their care. Indeed, spiritual care was central to the deaconess's work.

When the deaconesses identified opportunities to bring people together for a common purpose, they mobilized available resources and formally organized committees or groups in churches or at the motherhouse. On October 3, 1896, Eyster documented, "Help to organize a sewing school at Calvary church."[34] With unemployment found as a frequent complaint in the homes visited, the deaconesses often identified "impure surroundings" prompting the deaconess to invite the girls to the motherhouse once a month to form a "King's Daughter Circle which will be of help in many ways."[35] In creating the "Circle," the deaconesses worked to establish healthy relationships with young girls encouraging them to make good choices while also providing useful service in

---

[31]Lucy Eyster, *Pocket Notes 1896–1924*, ELCAA, ELCA 127/6/1, Deceased Personnel Files, 1884–2003, box 11, folder 9.

[32]Jennie Christ, *Daybook No. 5: Journeys Happy and Joyful*, ELCAA, ELCA 127/6/1 Deceased Personnel Files, box 8, quote from December 15, 1897.

[33]Eyster, *Pocket Notes*. See also, Christ, *Daybook No. 5*; Shaffer, *Daily Record of Events*, 5.

[34]Eyster, *Pocket Notes*, quote from October 3, 1896.

[35]Ibid., 5.

the community. Teaching children and modeling desired Christian behaviors was another form of visible deaconess work in the community.

The deaconess women were warmly welcomed into the homes of other women. Frequently, the deaconesses referred unemployed women capable of work to the King's Daughter Society and to families requesting domestic help in their homes.[36] The deaconesses were also known for enlisting persons to assist with motherhouse tasks such as cooking, ironing, and cleaning.[37] Eyster wrote on June 14, 1898, "Mrs. B., Find them getting along all right. Cora needs shoes. Tell Mrs. she can earn them at our house."[38] Where possible, the deaconesses identified opportunities for useful work in service to others. It was evident that social care was an integral component of the deaconess work in Baltimore.

Parish deaconesses understood the role of physicians during this period. In several instances while making home visits, the deaconess worked with physicians and received orders for patient care. Mutual recognition of one another's work is expressed in this deaconess diary entry dated December 15, 1897: "I found the Dr. who seemed glad that I had come to help him. He told me my patient had pneumonia and was very sick. Having left his orders he went home and after everything had been arranged for the night. . . . I tried to do all I could for my friend."[39]

The parish deaconess became a known and trusted resource for a congregation. In most cases after a few short months, the pastor and members of a congregation were convinced of the need for a parish deaconess. The members of St. John's Lutheran Church in Baltimore were candid in their description of the parish deaconess sent to them "whose whole soul was in the work . . . [and whose] cheerful face and hopeful spirit changed the outlook of the church both for the pastor and people."[40] In just 1 year, the parish deaconess documented "a thousand calls in the homes of the congregation and five hundred additional visits to the sick and needy . . . she nursed altogether eighteen families and did a lot of general work besides."[41] As part of the annual report to the congregation and to the motherhouse, the pastor spoke of how he could depend upon the deaconess to "always do her part, and as the work developed, [the pastor] allowed her largely to use her own judgment and good sense in going where she was most needed."[42] Thus, once the parish deaconess

---

[36]Shaffer, *Daily Record of Events,* quote from March 4, 1896, p. 8.
[37]Eyster, *Pocket Notes*, quote from March 24, 1896, p. 8.
[38]Eyster, *Pocket Notes*, quote from June 14, 1898.
[39]Christ, *Daybook No. 5*, quote from December 15, 1897.
[40]Freas, *The Parish Deaconess,* 4.
[41]Ibid., 7.
[42]Ibid., 7.

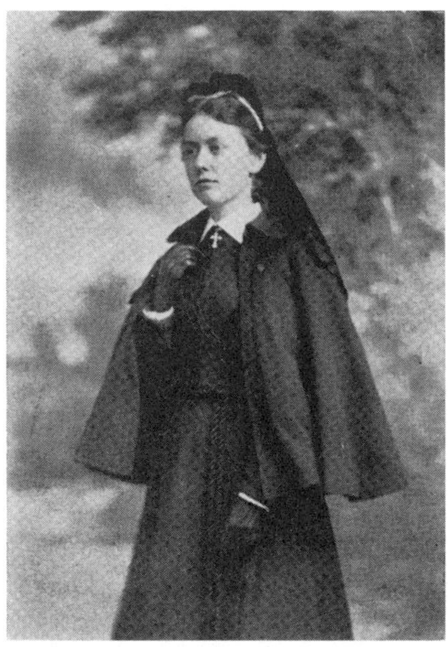

FIGURE 7.7 Sister Jennie Christ as a parish deaconess, ca. 1900. *Reprinted with permission of The Evangelical Lutheran Church in America Archives (Elk Grove Village, IL).*

proved her competency and skill, the clergy gave her permission to be more autonomous in her practice. Nonetheless, in the same annual report, the pastor hinted at gendered differences in ministry, noting that the women who served as parish deaconesses "have a way of seeing through things, though they may get little credit for it."[43]

In December 1897, Jennie Christ arrived on assignment to St. Luke's Parish of York, Pennsylvania. In this diary entry, Christ provides a summary of her work and her personal aspirations to care for those in need:

> Many and interesting have been my new experiences in a parish almost on the outskirts of a city. One finds a variety of services among the people. There are poor, there are sick, there are those who have become indifferent and those who seem to have not desire for the higher life and for a soul culture as a preparation for the life to come. Little did I think that I would ever be sent out as a parish deaconess. But every year brings new developments and brings with it oft times that which we least expect. God grant that some good may come out of the work which I have done here. In the weeks I have been here I have visited all of the members of the Church and Sunday School.[44]

---

[43]Ibid., 4.

[44]Christ, *Daybook No. 5*, quote from December 15, 1897.

Lutheran church leaders recognized that the Baltimore Motherhouse produced highly trained workers particularly adapted to the demands of the Lutheran congregation, and requests for parish deaconesses multiplied.[45] Parish deaconesses trained at Baltimore were sent out on assignments regionally and to multiple locations outside of Baltimore. Documented in the 1903 Motherhouse handbook, approximately 20 consecrated parish deaconesses who wore the Lutheran garb and Baltimore deaconess cross were sent as far away as Richmond, Indiana, and Cincinnati, Ohio. Deaconesses were assigned to Maryland congregations in Baltimore and in Cumberland and then to cities in Pennsylvania and New York.[46] Altogether, over an 8-year period, Baltimore parish deaconesses served 100 parishes with nearly 80 pastors and in more than 1,000 homes of Lutheran parishioners. Ultimately, the parish deaconesses assigned to congregations complemented the work of the pastor and augmented the social ministry initiatives of each congregation. Collectively, the Baltimore parish deaconesses promoted a community model of wholistic care addressing unmet physical, social, and spiritual needs.

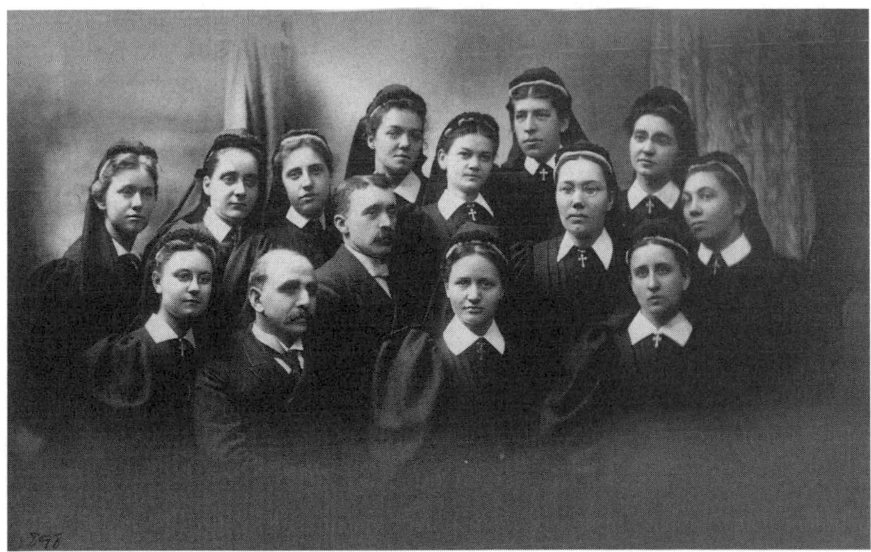

FIGURE 7.8 Portrait of deaconesses wearing garb including Baltimore Motherhouse cross of consecration with motherhouse pastors, ca. 1898. *Reprinted with permission of The Evangelical Lutheran Church in America Archives (Elk Grove Village, IL).*

---

[45]Nicholas, *The Pastor and the Deaconess*, 1.

[46]BDM, *Handbook: Lutheran Deaconess Motherhouse and Training School 1903* (Baltimore, MD: Lutheran Deaconess Motherhouse, n.d., ELCAA, ULCA 61/8/1, Handbook/Catalogue, Lutheran Deaconess Motherhouse and Training School, 1895, 1903–1947, box 1, folder 1: 23–25).

IMPLICATIONS FOR NURSING PRACTICE TODAY

The Lutheran deaconess history challenges current assumptions about nursing and healthcare. First, in addition to addressing individual's physical and emotional needs, there is a need to reclaim the spiritual dimension of nursing regardless of care setting. This recognizes that the spirit is the core of the person and the person cannot be separated from his or her spiritual self.[47] With chronic disease and unhealthy lifestyle choices continuing to challenge available resources today, wholistic care is relevant for nursing practice whether engaged in faith-based initiatives such as parish nursing or working in secular healthcare.

Second, health systems are challenged to promote whole-person care. While healthcare providers, including nurses, are aware of the benefits of providing wholistic care to patients, often the primary focus is on the physical aspect of care coupled with a hesitancy to address spiritual care needs particularly in secular settings. In an effort to encourage wholistic care for patients, The Joint Commission requires accredited hospitals to make provision for a patient's spiritual care needs during encounters with healthcare personnel, including nurses, regardless of setting.[48] Thus, all patients should receive a standard of care addressing the whole person—body, mind, and spirit. Since hospitals routinely provide episodic illness care and do not have the time or resources to establish long-term relationships allowing for health promotion and healing, creative initiatives across the continuum of care involving hospital chaplains, parish nurses, and community clergy are a necessity.

Finally, it is important for faith communities to restore a healing mission for their membership. The faith community may be the only institution that interacts with a person from birth through death. Thus, there is great opportunity for a nurse working out of the congregational setting to promote health

---

[47]Kristen L. Mauk, "The Role of the Nurse in the Spiritual Journey," in *Spiritual Care in Nursing Practice*, eds. Kristen L. Mauk and Nola K. Schmidt (Philadelphia, PA: Lippincott Williams & Wilkins, 2004), 190.

[48]The Joint Commission, *Comprehensive Accreditation Manual for Hospitals: The Official Handbook* (Chicago, IL: Joint Commission Resources, 2009), 1. The Joint Commission is responsible for the accreditation of healthcare institutions and mandates standards of care for quality, safety, and individual-centered healthcare. The Patient Rights and Organization Ethics standard 2.10 entitled *Ethics, Rights and Responsibilities* is specific to spiritual care for patients and requires the hospital to accommodate the patient's right to religious and other spiritual services.

and provide wholistic care to persons across the lifespan serving as a complement to any supportive care of family members and the pastor's ministry. Indeed, the faith community provides an ideal setting for a registered nurse to become the known and trusted faith community nurse promoting health, healing, and wholeness.[49]

ACKNOWLEDGMENTS

Special thanks to Drs. Arlene Keeling and Barbara Brodie of the University of Virginia's Center for Nursing Historical Inquiry for encouraging and supporting scholarly research in nursing history.

---

[49]Granger E. Westberg, *Typed Paper Describing the Role of the PN (circa 1985–86)*, from personal collection of Phyllis Ann Solari-Twadell accessed March 2006. See also American Nurses and Health Ministries Association, Inc., *Scope and Standards of Parish Nursing Practice*, (Washington, DC: American Nurses Association, 1998), 1. The contemporary faith-based nursing movement known as *parish nursing* began in 1984 with the work of Lutheran chaplain, Granger Westberg. He observed that a nurse working out of the congregational setting is in a unique position to promote wholistic care of body, mind, and spirit. In defining the parish nurse role, Westberg borrowed from his experience with interdisciplinary Wholistic Health Centers located in congregations and the work of nineteenth-century religious nurses, both Catholic and Protestant, in Europe and America. Parish nursing is recognized as a specialty practice by the American Nurses Association, and is defined as: "a professional nursing [role] that focuses on the intentional care of the spirit as part of the process of promoting wholistic health and preventing or minimizing illness in a faith community."

Section III

NURSING INTERVENTIONS: INFLUENCING CHANGE

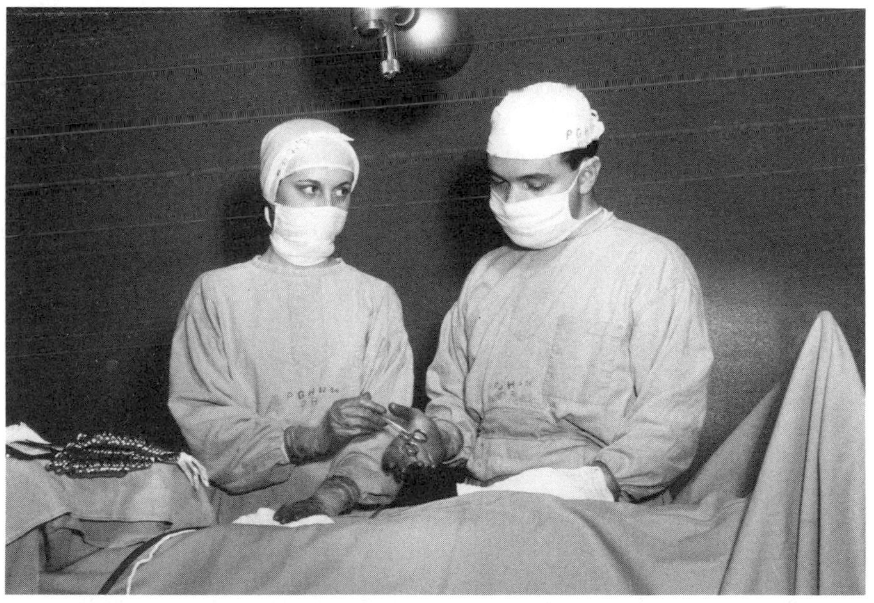

Nurse and doctor in the operating room of the Philadelphia General Hospital, ca. 1954. *Reprinted with permission of the Barbara Bates Center for the Study of the History of Nursing.*

CHAPTER 8

Obstetric Nursing: For the Patient or the Doctor?

Sylvia Rinker

INTRODUCTION

It is a scene familiar in birthing units in hospitals across America. The expectant mother and her partner arrive in breathless anticipation of the birth of their long-planned-for and well-scheduled baby. After thoroughly researching all of their options, the couple decide that the safest place to have their baby is in the hospital, primarily because emergency equipment, medication, oxygen, and medical personnel will be readily available should something happen to either the mother or the baby. They intend to maintain control over their birthing process, however, and have brought with them a detailed birth plan that outlines their preferences about pain relief and other interventions during their labor and delivery. Conventional wisdom among experienced staff is that it is precisely the mother who will try to manage labor without pain relief, will fail, will eventually receive epidural anesthesia, and finally because of fetal distress or other problem, will undergo a cesarean section. Nurses who function within this pattern are reaping the legacy of scientific birth, ushered into the hospital by nurses who were specially chosen by doctors in the early 1900s to convince mothers that medical care with its interventions for birth was a modern, safe, and scientific idea.

Physician-attended hospitalized birth, with all of its inherent interventions, has become entrenched in American society. In 2006, 99% of all births in America were in hospitals, with 91.5% of those delivered by physicians.[1] Unfortunately, the promise of safer birth when attended by specialist physicians has fallen short. Despite maternity care delivered almost exclusively by specialists in hospitals, the maternal mortality rate in the United States remains at 15 deaths per 100,000 live births, far from the Healthy People 2010 target of 3 deaths per 100,000.[2] Further frustrating those who care for mothers in America is that despite spending more on healthcare per person than any other nation in the world, maternal mortality rates in the United States were higher than those in 33 other countries in 2005.[3] Current debates about the urgency of healthcare reform highlight the conundrum that has placed the process of birth, a generally healthy, low-risk event, almost entirely within the confines of expensive hospital care. Efforts to establish best practices based on evidence-based care have produced a wealth of research, but unfortunately not yet produced the outcomes desired. The Milbank Memorial Fund's recent publication "Evidence-Based Maternity Care: What It Is and What It Can Achieve" offers the troubling conclusion that despite good intentions and large expenditures of money, the U.S. maternity care system is failing to provide the safe outcomes for mothers and infants that medical science promised at the outset of the twentieth century.[4] As key players in the care of pregnant women, nurses share both the credit and the blame for the current situation. What evidence might there be for current practice as revealed in the historical outcomes thus far?

Investigation into the evolution of obstetric nursing clinical practice offers insight into the conflict between science and nurturing that erupted as nursing ideals confronted the everyday experiences of the nurses and patients

---

[1]Joyce Martin, Brady Hamilton, Paul Sutton, Stephanie Ventura, Fay Menacker, Sharon Kirmeyer, and T. J. Mathews, Division of Vital Statistics, Centers for Disease Control and Prevention, "Births: Final Data for 2006," *National Vital Statistics Reports* 57 (January 7, 2009): 16, http://www.cdc.gov/nchs/data/nvsr/nvsr57/nvsr57_07.pdf (accessed October 10, 2009).

[2]Joint Commission, "Safer Pregnancies: Improving Maternal Mortality Rates," *Joint Commission Benchmark* 11 (January/February 2009): 4.

[3]Childbirth Connection, "Maternity Quality Matters," *Childbirth Connection* (2009), http://www.childbirthconnection.org/article.asp?ck=10574&ClickedLink=919&area=27 (accessed October 10 2009). Childbirth Connection is a national not-for-profit organization founded in 1918 as the Maternity Center Association in New York to combat maternal mortality.

[4]Carol Sakala and Maureen Corry, *Evidence-Based Maternity Care: What It Is and What It Can Achieve* (New York: Milbank Memorial Fund, 2008).

involved.[5] Tensions between the nurse's role as a scientific manager and her expected function as a nurturing caregiver were evident at the outset of professional nursing; a century later the conflict between providing care as dictated by medical science and the supportive care laboring patients need remains unresolved.[6] The clinical practice nurses developed, viewed as an outcome of choices made in the past, offers insight into the continuing ambiguity of the historical role of nurses expected to function as both scientific and caring practitioners.[7]

RECRUITMENT OF THE NURSE

Literature of the early decades of the twentieth century clearly and repeatedly proclaimed that woman's primary responsibilities resided in the home; her most lauded roles were those of wife and mother. Then, the characteristics of piety, domesticity, purity, and submissiveness defined "true womanhood."[8] From colonial days, female midwives had been the expected and accepted attendants for births occurring at home, where female friends and relatives came to provide comfort and practical aid to the expectant mother and her family.[9] Midwives practicing in the early 1900s gained their knowledge of childbirth in formal training schools in the European or Asian countries of their birth, or from experience passed down from generation to generation without formal education.

---

[5]Sylvia Rinker, "To Cultivate a Feeling of Confidence: The Nursing of Obstetric Patients, 1890–1940," *Nursing History Review* 8 (2000): 117–142. Portions of this article are reprinted here with permission from Springer Publishing.

[6]Elaine Hodnett, Nancy Lowe, Mary Hannah et al., "Effectiveness of Nurses as Providers of Birth Labor Support in North American Hospitals," *Journal of American Medical Association* 288 (September 18, 2002): 1373–1381; Elaine Zwelling, "The Emergence of High-Tech Birthing," *Journal of Obstetric, Gynecological, and Neonatal Nursing* 37 (January 2008): 85–93; Alison Kitson, "Does Nursing Have a Future?" *Image* 29 (Second Quarter 1997): 111–115.

[7]Charles Rosenberg, "Clio and Caring: An Agenda for American Historians and Nursing," *Nursing Research* 26 (January/February 1987): 67–68.

[8]See Barbara Welter, "The Cult of True Womanhood: 1820–1860," *American Quarterly* 18 (Summer 1966): 151–174; Linda Kerber, "Separate Spheres, Female Worlds, Woman's Place: The Rhetoric of Women's History," *The Journal of American History* 75 (June 1988): 9–39, for discussions of the ideology of "true womanhood" and its popular components of piety, purity, domesticity, and submissiveness. The preface to *The Perfect Woman* clearly delineated woman's primary function, cautioning its readers that "While we admire (the woman) in her new role, with her efforts towards success in society, literature, science, politics, and the arts, we must not lose sight of her most divine and sublime mission in life—womanhood and motherhood." Mary Melendy, *The Perfect Woman* (K.T. Boland, 1903), 7.

[9]Richard Wertz and Dorothy Wertz, *Lying-In: A History of Childbirth in America*, expanded ed. (New Haven, CT: Yale University Press, 1989), 2.

Irrespective of their backgrounds, their practice of delivering mothers without the benefit of medical oversight threatened the credibility of the newly emerging obstetric medical science.[10] Nurse-midwives did not practice until the 1930s.[11] The "trained nurse" identifier separated the woman who had received scientific education from just any woman whose innate characteristics were assumed to equip her to care for the sick. Recruited because she was a woman, the newly emerging "trained nurse"[12] was charged with the task of convincing women to abandon the familiar female-surrounded birth-at-home experience attended by lay midwives in favor of the rapidly growing scientific medical childbirth in the hospital.[13] "Filling the gap between home and hospital adequately" and "smoothing the path for the obstetric art" were duties that the nurse, as an educated early twentieth-century woman, was deemed qualified to perform.[14]

The concerted efforts by physicians to discredit midwives eventually succeeded in their near elimination. While in 1900 midwives delivered 50% of births, by 1930, they delivered only 15%, and by 1973, this figure had dropped to less than 1%.[15] Physicians and others championed nurses as assistants at birth instead of midwives because nurses accepted a position that was clearly subordinate to that of the physician. The nurse's role was as an *assistant* to the physician, not as a substitute. The dilemma this created for nursing was that rather than medicine and nursing developing as separate but complementary professions with a shared focus on patient care, nursing was defined as the work of a subordinate group

---

[10]Specific efforts by physicians trying to win prestige and recognition for the obstetric specialty included eliminating competitors, upgrading the standards of medical education and practice, and linking forces with the surgical specialty of gynecology. Nancy Dye, "The Medicalization of Birth," in *The American Way of Birth,* ed. Pamela Eakins, (Philadelphia, PA: Temple University Press, 1986).

[11]Charlotte Borst, *Catching Babies: The Professionalization of Childbirth, 1870–1920* (Cambridge, MA: Harvard University Press, 1995).

[12]Nurses were educated and practiced as generalists; the term "obstetric nurse" was the title given to the nurse who cared for obstetric patients. Herbert Stowe, "The Specially Trained Obstetric Nurse—Her Advantages and Her Field," *American Journal of Nursing* 10 (May 1910): 550–554.

[13]R. Wertz and D.Wertz, *Lying-In*; Judith Leavitt, *Brought to Bed: Childbearing in America 1750–1950* (New York: Oxford University Press, 1986); Nancy Dye, "Modern Obstetrics and Working-Class Women: The New York Midwifery Dispensary, 1890–1920," *Journal of Social History* 20 (1987): 549–564.

[14]Joseph B. DeLee, *Obstetrics for Nurses,* 2nd ed. (Philadelphia, PA: W.B. Saunders, 1907), 18; Joseph B. DeLee, "The Prophylactic Forceps Operation," *American Journal of Obstetrics and Gynecology* 1 (1920): 34–44.

[15]White House Conference on Child Health and Protection, *Obstetric Education* (New York: The Century, 1931), 169; William McCool and Sandi McCool, "Feminism and Nurse-Midwifery: Historical Overview and Current Issues," *Journal of Nurse Midwifery* 34 (November/December 1989): 323–334.

whose emphasis was not improved patient care, but rather improved medical practice. In this scheme, the clear priority was assisting the physician and promoting medical practice; comforting the patient took second place.

Joseph B. DeLee, a dominant figure in American obstetrics at the turn of the twentieth century, prescribed a specific role for the nurse explicitly designed to benefit the new obstetric "specialty" and its physician practitioners.[16] He said:

> The nurse may do much to aid the physician in obtaining from the public that recognition for obstetrics that the specialty so justly deserves. Thus, the nurse may smooth the path for the advance of the obstetric art. She becomes really a missionary spreading the gospel of good obstetrics.[17]

As defined by the influential DeLee, childbirth required that strict limits, imposed by scientific asepsis rules, be applied to nursing practice. Thus, from the outset, the nurse's innate female attributes, governed by the scientific principles of obstetric medicine, constituted the foundations for both the power and the limits of obstetric nursing. Welcoming the status afforded by their association with the newly emerging specialist-obstetricians, nurses readily accepted a role they were only partially able to define. Charged with delivering scientific care, nurses remained on the periphery in defining the dimensions of that care.[18]

NURSES AND PHYSICIANS: A USEFUL ALLIANCE

The belief in the power of science held by early twentieth-century Americans to improve the lives of citizens and the growing power of the medical profession made the association of nursing with medicine an attractive alliance to nurse-leaders.[19] Eager to promote nursing as a respectable profession, Isabel Hampton referred to the nurse as the "physician's lieutenant," who, by virtue of her

---

[16]Joseph B. DeLee was born in 1869 and died in 1942. He authored 100 articles, 18 editions of *Obstetrics for Nurses* beginning in 1904, and 13 editions of *The Principles and Practice of Obstetrics*, first published in 1913. He founded the Maxwell Street Dispensary and Chicago Lying-In Hospital in 1895. By the time of his death in 1942, he had well earned his reputation as a "formidable force in American obstetrics." Judith Leavitt, "Joseph B. DeLee and the Practice of Preventive Obstetrics," *American Journal of Public Health* 78 (October 1988): 1353–1360.
[17]DeLee, *Obstetrics for Nurses*, 18; DeLee, "The Prophylactic Forceps Operation," 34–44.
[18]DeLee, *Obstetrics for Nurses*; Herbert Stowe, "The Specially Trained Obstetric Nurse—Her Advantages and Field," *American Journal of Nursing* 10 (1910): 550.
[19]Robert Wiebe, *The Search for Order: 1877–1920* (New York: Hill and Wang, 1967); Judith Leavitt, "Science Enters the Birthing Room: Obstetrics in America Since the Eighteenth Century," *Journal of American History* 70 (September 1983): 303.

training, was "allotted a part to perform in the progress of medical science."[20] Hampton's vision of the possibilities for nursing included a clear commitment to standards, precision, and method for the organization, teaching, and practice of nursing.[21] Speaking at the Chicago World's Fair in 1893, and demonstrating her understanding that working within the system could strengthen the position of the nursing profession, Hampton willingly accepted a limited role for nurses, as she said: "To be sure, the nurse is only the handmaid of that great and beautiful medical science in whose temple she may only serve in minor parts."[22]

Anxious to establish themselves as valuable assistants to physicians, nurses developed a practice that gave priority to medical science and the needs of physicians over the needs of individual patients. Scientific principles provided the foundation for the beginning practice of obstetric nursing and directly affected the relationships nurses established with their patients. Georgina Pope, Superintendent of Nurses at the Columbia Hospital for Women in Washington, DC, underscored the central role of the nurse and her value as a scientific practitioner when she said:

> It is through the nurse that the doctor expects to combat the frightful disease of puerperal fever . . . she can become of no less importance than the physician himself in guarding the health and preserving the lives of mothers and children.[23]

THE PROMISE OF SAFE AND PAINLESS DELIVERIES

Certainly the life-threatening danger of puerperal sepsis colored the evolution of obstetric nursing. Oliver Wendell Holmes, dean of the Harvard Medical School, was a well-known poet, author, and medical researcher who published the classic article "On the Contagiousness of Puerperal Fever," in 1843.[24] By 1879, Louis Pasteur had demonstrated that the infectious streptococcus was

---

[20]Isabel Hampton, "Educational Standards for Nurses," in *Nursing of the Sick 1893: Papers and Discussions from the International Congress of Charities, Corrections, and Philanthropy, Chicago 1893* (New York: National League of Nursing Education, 1949).

[21]Ellen Baer, "Nursing's Divided House—An Historical View," *Nursing Research* 34 (January/February 1985): 32–38.

[22]Hampton, "Educational Standards for Nurses," 2.

[23]Georgina Pope, "Obstetric Nursing," in *Nursing of the Sick 1893: Papers and Discussions from the International Congress of Charities, Corrections, and Philanthropy, Chicago 1893* (New York: National League of Nursing Education, 1949), 166.

[24]Oliver Wendell Holmes, "On the Contagiousness of Puerperal Fever," *New England Quarterly Journal of Medicine and Surgery* 6 (1842–1843): 503–530.

responsible for puerperal fever.[25] Science had provided a way, through antiseptic and aseptic practices, to overcome the killer, and its principles must *not* be violated. In 1924, Charles Reed, an influential physician practicing obstetrics in Illinois was invited to speak at the annual meeting of the Illinois State Association of Graduate Nurses. He identified the "foundational qualities" of the nurse to be courage, tenderness, and self-control—but there was more:

> and yet, though she have the courage of a lioness, the divine tenderness of a mother, and the self-control of a Capulet, and have not science, it shall profit her nothing. Her training in science, science clear, precise, inevitable, is the necessary medium through which her mind and emotions express themselves. It is the master tool of her profession.[26]

The traditional nursing values of compassion, comfort, and support for the whole person clashed with the rigors of scientific asepsis that defined the medical practice of obstetrics; the nursing care that developed bore the marks of this conflict.

Once the public had been convinced to accept medical attendance at birth, the womanly attributes of the nurse were redirected to support physicians and medical procedures rather than the patient who was giving birth. As good missionaries, obstetric nurses believed the gospel that strict adherence to asepsis principles was requisite to save the lives of mothers and babies. As there could be no tolerance for breaks in aseptic technique, there could be no deviation in the hospital routine that might permit the introduction of the infectious germ. The hard-fought battle against maternal mortality was just beginning to lower the death rates of mothers in the late 1930s, and, despite patients' complaints, nurses were convinced that the rigid hospital policies were justified to protect their patients.

OPERATIVE INTERVENTIONS FOR BIRTH

The hospitalization of birth facilitated a greater number and frequency of procedures that greatly increased nurses' duties, further securing their position within the hospital. From 1890 to 1940, a dramatic increase in the "operative interventions" used for childbirth in hospitals is clearly evident. The use of forceps,

---

[25]See Elaine Larson, "Innovations in Health Care: Antisepsis as a Case Study," *American Journal of Public Health* 79 (January 1989): 92–99, for a complete discussion of the controversy over the contagiousness of puerperal fever in the mid-nineteenth century.

[26]Charles Reed, "Teaching Obstetrics to Student Nurses," *American Journal of Nursing* 24 (December 1924): 1210–1211. Quote is on p. 1211.

mechanical induction, versions, episiotomies, and cesarean sections had all been available since the mid-nineteenth century, but their use exploded as the twentieth century progressed.[27] The overall operative intervention rate for deliveries at Columbia Hospital in Washington, DC, for example, more than tripled from 20% in 1892 to 66% in 1920.[28] Sixty-five percent of the women who delivered at the Chicago Lying-In Hospital between 1918 and 1925 had operative deliveries; by 1931, 80% of women received some type of intervention for birth.[29]

Rigid routines were developed to streamline the extra care required by the growing population of hospitalized patients who were receiving increasing numbers of interventions for their births. Physicians lent their authority and nurses used it willingly to promote scientific birth restrictions. Asepsis rules required banning family and friends from the laboring rooms in the hospitals. Nurses willingly supported policies that separated a woman from her family on her admission to the hospital, stripped her of her clothes, shaved her, purged her, and sometimes restrained her, all in the pursuit of asepsis.[30] Individualized care suffered under this regime and certainly contributed to the dissatisfaction among mothers that Leavitt has documented.[31] The nurses who participated in such actions believed the scientific training they had received; they were convinced that such policies were justified to save mothers and infants from death.

---

[27]Mechanical induction involved the use of inflatable balloons pushed through the cervix or other instruments to forcibly dilate the cervix. Janet Ashford, "A History of Accouchement Force," *Birth* 13 (December 1986): 241–249. Version was a method of turning the infant in the uterus for a more favorable presentation for birth. Stephen Thacker and David Banta, "Benefits and Risks of Episiotomy: An Interpretive Review of the English Language Literature, 1860–1980," *Obstetrical and Gynecological Survey* 38 (1983): 322–338; Jane Sewell, *Cesarean Section—A Brief History* (Washington, DC: American College of Obstetricians and Gynecologists, 1993).

[28]*Annual Reports of the Columbia Hospital for Women: 1800–1920*, located in the hospital administrator's office, Columbia Hospital for Women and Medical Center, Washington, DC.

[29]*Statistical Report of the Chicago Lying-In Hospital and Dispensary, 1918–1925; 1925–1927; and 1928–1931*, Lying-In Hospital Records Collection, University of Chicago Library, Chicago, Illinois.

[30]Bernice Gardner, "Nursing Care During the Administration of Rectal Anesthesia," *American Journal of Nursing* 31 (July 1921): 794–798; C.O. McCormick, "Rectal Ether Analgesia in Obstetrics," American Journal of Nursing 33 (May 1933): 415–422. Anne Yelton and Marie Hilgediek, "Rectal Ether Analgesia from the Nurse's Standpoint," *American Journal of Nursing* 33 (May 1933): 420–422; Harold H. Rosenfield, "Analgesia in Obstetrics," *American Journal of Nursing* 35 (May 1935): 437–440; Catherine Yeo, "Technic of Administration [Analgesia in Obstetrics] and Nursing Care," *American Journal of Nursing* 35 (May 1935): 440–442; Margarete Sandelowski, *Pain, Pleasure and American Childbirth* (Westport, CT: Greenwood Press, 1984).

[31]Judith Leavitt, "Strange Young Women on Errands: Obstetric Nursing Between Two Worlds," *Nursing History Review* 6 (1998): 3–24.

Second only to the fear of death in childbirth among women, at the end of the nineteenth century was a nearly universal dread of pain.[32] American women actively sought anesthesia, offered as one of the chief advantages of scientific birth.[33] Registered nurse Mary Blackwell understood the challenge and the prestige of nursing the medicated woman in labor when she observed in 1931 that "the nursing care of obstetric patients having analgesia and anesthesia is a difficult, though interesting duty."[34] The nurse administered the medication and applied the restraints, changing in the process, as historian Margarete Sandelowski has noted, "from a sisterly companion to an unfeeling robot."[35] Birth became an event not to be accepted and celebrated, but one to be managed and controlled. Because the anesthetized, restless patient could give no warning of an impending birth, making precipitous delivery very likely, the nurse who managed such a process successfully was obviously an essential facilitator of scientific birth.

CONFLICT: MANAGING THE SYSTEM AND SUSTAINING THE PATIENT

Charged with spreading the gospel of good obstetrics, nurses first discovered that their management skills were necessary in homes to keep the household functioning during the disruption caused by application of the required asepsis principles for scientific birth.[36] As managers in the hospitals, nurses were also responsible to promote the smooth, efficient running of the institution. Nurses became adept at the scientific management of equipment, personnel, patients, and families in the hospitals. The priority for nursing care was to "smooth the path" for the physician, followed closely by efforts to ensure the economic efficiency of the hospital.

As hospitals changed from charity institutions to business enterprises, efficiency was prized for its economic value as well as for its influence on the

---

[32]Wertz and Wertz, *Lying-In*; Sandelowski, *Pain, Pleasure and American Childbirth;* Sylvia Hoffert, *Private Matters: American Attitudes Toward Childbearing and Infant Nurture in the Urban North, 1800-1860* (Urbana, IL: University of Illinois Press, 1989).

[33]Leavitt, *Brought to Bed*. See especially Chapter 5: "The Greatest Blessing of This Age," Pain Relief in Obstetrics.

[34]Mary Blackwell, "The Nursing Care of Obstetric Patients Having Analgesia and Anesthesia," *American Journal of Nursing* 33 (May 1933): 425–427; Pierce Rucker, "Obstetric Analgesia and Anesthesia," *American Journal of Nursing* 33 (May 1933): 423–425.

[35]Sandelowski, *Pain, Pleasure, and American Childbirth*, 68.

[36]M. McCullough, "A Normal Home Delivery," *Trained Nurse and Hospital Review* 102 (1939): 419–424.

happiness of physicians.[37] Beginning in the 1920s, caught in an ever-greater push for hospital efficiency and economy, nurses participated in time–motion studies of nursing procedures and divided nursing care into component parts.[38] In the process, the sympathetic, womanly qualities, so crucial for the acceptance of medical birth, were submerged under a scientific mold that required conformity and a standardized approach to patient care. Nurses developed and published clearly delineated standards and procedures in professional journals that reflected the values of the developing profession. Detailed drawings in texts and journals showed *the* correct way to bind the abdomen and breasts following birth, *the* correct way to place instruments on a perineal care tray, and outlined strict schedules for maternal and infant elimination and feeding.[39] As they developed nursing procedures, questions about the relative merits of various solutions used for perineal care, about the most efficient breast care, and questions about what was the quickest way, compatible with safety and comfort, of getting 20 bedpans to 20 patients were all of concern to the developing professional nurses in the 1930s.[40] Articles published in journals of the time show that nurses were beginning to follow the medical model of scientific research to validate nursing interventions. As nursing progressed, documenting the contributions of nurses to medical practice was a first step, necessary for the acknowledgment of nurses as skilled professionals. In the evolution of nursing, expertise in the application of scientific medical knowledge was foundational for the future recognition of nursing as a legitimate profession.

---

[37]Charles Rosenberg, *The Care of Strangers* (New York: Basic Books, 1987), and Rosemary Stevens, *In Sickness and in Wealth: American Hospitals in the Twentieth Century* (New York: Basic Books, 1989).

[38]Chelly Wasserberg and Ethel Northam, "Some Time Studies in Obstetrical Nursing," *American Journal of Nursing* 27 (July 1927): 543–544; Lillian S. Clayton, "Standardizing Nursing Technic: Its Advantages and Disadvantages," *American Journal of Nursing* 27 (November 1927): 939–943.

[39]Nellie Brown, "A Movable Perineal Dressing Tray," *American Journal of Nursing* 24 (November 1924): 875–876; Mildred Newton, "The Noiseless Perineal Dressing Cart," *American Journal of Nursing* 28 (July 1928): 667–668; M. Cordelia Cowen, "A Study of Breast Care: Part I," *American Journal of Nursing* 29 (October 1929): 1165–1170; Cowen, "A Study of Breast Care: Part II," *American Journal of Nursing* 29 (November 1929): 1299–1306; DeLee, *Obstetrics for Nurses*; Clara Weeks-Shaw, *Textbook of Nursing*, 3rd ed. (New York: Appleton, 1912); Louise Zabriskie, *Nurses Handbook of Obstetrics*, 1st through 6th eds. (Philadelphia, PA: J.B. Lippincott, 1929, 1931, 1933, 1934, 1937, and 1940); Carolyn Van Blarcom, *Obstetrical Nursing*, 2nd ed. (New York: Macmillan, 1932).

[40]Emily Shaffer, "Perineal Technic," *American Journal of Nursing* 34 (January 1934): 26–28; "A Survey of Methods Used in Four Hospitals," *American Journal of Nursing* 31 (March 1931): 313–317; Joyce Roberts, "Maternal Positions for Childbirth: A Historical Review of Nursing Care Practices," *Journal of Obstetric, Gynecologic, and Neonatal Nursing* 8 (January/February 1979): 24–32.

But as both nurses and patients soon realized, the purely scientific approach, while accepted as necessary, was insufficient to meet patients' needs.[41]

THE NURSE'S POINT OF VIEW

By 1940, nurses who worked in specific labor and delivery, postpartum, and nursery units began to develop a clinical expertise and familiarity with the routine that freed them to pay attention to patients' needs for comfort beyond the strict scientific application of medical treatments. In the process of smoothing the path for the advance of obstetrics, nurses had begun to develop a vision no longer confined to the field of medicine. While cooperative with medicine, nursing was moving beyond a physician definition of the function of nurses. Nurses lent their energy, intelligence, and abilities to promote medical care for childbirth, but because of their relationships with patients, nurses were privileged to a particular kind of knowledge that, while derived from and complementary to medical knowledge, was different. As the profession grew, nurses used their insights to shape nursing practice; the missionary began to craft her own message. Carolyn Van Blarcom, one of the first nurses to write an obstetric nursing textbook, clearly stated: "Asepsis must come first and foremost, but the nurse's attitude and care of her patient must be mellowed by an always deepening sympathy and understanding." She continued:

> Good nursing implies more than the giving of bed baths and medicines, boiling instruments and serving meals. It is more than going on duty at a certain time, carrying out orders for a certain number of hours and going off duty again. It implies care and consideration of the patient as a human being and a determination to nurse her well and happily, no matter what this demands.[42]

Using their knowledge and experience to discuss patient care, nurses began, formally, to define and develop nursing procedures.

WHAT TO DO WITH THE EVIDENCE?

The trend of increasing interventions has continued into the twenty-first century.[43] Induction, the practice of starting labor with medications, rose from 9.5% of births in 1990 to 20% of births since 1999. A 20-year survey

---

[41]Leavitt, "Strange Young Women on Errands."
[42]Van Blarcom, *Obstetrical Nursing,* 5.
[43]CDC, US Department of Health and Human Services, "Births: Final Data for 2006," *National Vital Statistics Reports* 57 (January 7, 2009).

of obstetric anesthesia indicated a threefold increase in epidural anesthesia used for labor, from 22% in 1981 to 61% in 2001.[44] A "cascade of interventions" results when medications are used to induce labor causing strong, rapid contractions that then require epidural pain relief that then prohibits movement that then requires urinary catheterization that then exposes the mother to infection that also interferes with the mother's ability to push that ultimately requires a cesarean section delivery.[45] Although the World Health Organization recommends that the cesarean section rate should not be higher than 10% to 15%,[46] the cesarean section rate is currently more than 30% in the United States.[47]

Today's nurses face problems that in many ways are similar to those faced by their predecessors. The ambiguity of the nurse's role, conflicting loyalties, and the shifting structures of healthcare continue to complicate a clear definition of nursing responsibilities. Initially sought for their domestic abilities, nurses soon learned that scientific expertise gave them authority and prestige in the medical environment where they practiced.[48] As willing converts to the promises of science, the history of nurses and medical technology has been largely one of uncritical acceptance and integration into practice.[49] However, in light of the less-than-favorable outcomes of the routine use of technology such as electronic fetal monitoring during labor, some practicing nurses have begun to raise questions about the logic of the unquestioning adoption of

---

[44]Brenda Bucklin, Joy Hawkins, James Anderson, and Fred Ullrich, "Obstetric Anesthesia Workforce Survey: Twenty-year Update," *Anesthesiology* 103 (September 2005): 645–653.

[45]Childbirth Connection, "Cascade of Intervention in Childbirth," (September 4, 2009), http://www.childbirthconnection.org/article.asp?ck=10182 (accessed October 13, 2009).

[46]Nils Chaillet, Eric Dube, Marylene Dugas, Diane Francoeur, Johanne Dube, Sonia Gagnon, Lucie Poitras, and Alexandre Dumont, "Identifying Barriers and Facilitators Towards Implementing Guidelines to Reduce Caesarean Rates in Quebec," *Bulletin of the World Health Organization* 85 (October 2007): 733–820.

[47]Childbirth Connection, "Why Maternity Care Quality Matters," (September 2008). http://www.chilbirthconnection.org/article.asp?ck=10574&ClickedLink=919&area=27 (accessed October 13, 2009).

[48]Patricia D'Antonio has urged the recognition of nurses' domestic abilities as the source of their strength and power. Patricia O'Brien D'Antonio, "The Legacy of Domesticity: Nursing in Nineteenth Century America," *Nursing History Review* 1 (1993): 229–246.

[49]Margrete Sandelowski, "A Case of Conflicting Paradigms: Nursing and Reproductive Technology," *Advances in Nursing Science* 10 (1988): 35–45. Sandelowski has conducted extensive investigations into questions about the historical effects of technology on nursing care. See Sandelowski, "(Ir)Reconcilable Differences? The Debate Concerning Nursing and Technology," *Image* 29 (Second Quarter 1997): 169–174; "'Making the Best of Things': Technology in American Nursing, 1870–1940," *Nursing History Review* 5 (1997): 3–22.

such technology.[50] The current challenge in today's high-tech environment for birth seems to be a philosophical struggle between the desire to acknowledge and support birth as a normal event and the ever-growing perceived need for technology to provide state-of-the-art, safe care.[51]

The historical evidence is that nurses' skillful movements between their essential and ancillary positions successfully smoothed the path for obstetrics, but also contributed to their invisibility within the earliest healthcare systems. As a result, the nurturing relationship requisite for effective nursing and satisfied patients was also hidden, overlooked, and devalued. Historian Thomas Olson has documented that the "handling, managing, and controlling" abilities of students were the attributes praised by nursing superintendents between 1915 and 1937, while the "language of caring" was absent.[52] Historical evidence of the clinical outcomes, as real nurses translated ideal practices into the confines of everyday nursing, however, indicates that a fundamental source of nurses' power, knowledge, and influence, was found in the relationships they established with their patients.

Across the ages (and across cultures), new mothers and their families have consistently identified nursing support as a primary ingredient for their satisfaction with childbirth care.[53] The human person-to-person connection, so easily taken for granted, was at the core of effective nursing in the first half of this century. Nearly a century ago, nurse Sara Bower recognized the significance of nurse–patient relationships, when she identified as the nurse's *primary* duty "to cultivate at all times a feeling of confidence in the patient."[54]

The promises made by the emerging obstetric art in the early 1900s to address expectant mothers' twin fears at the turn of the century—the fear of death and the fear of pain—continue to be powerful motivators for new families to search out the best care available. Today, consumers of healthcare

---

[50]Kristen Priddy, "Is There Logic Behind Fetal Monitoring?" *Journal of Obstetric, Gynecologic, and Neonatal Nursing* 33 (September/October 2004): 550–553.

[51]Elaine Zwelling, "The Emergence of High-Tech Birthing," *Journal of Obstetric, Gynecologic, and Neonatal Nursing* 37 (2008): 85–93.

[52]Thomas Olson, "Laying Claim to Caring: Nursing and the Language of Training," *Nursing Outlook* 41 (March/April 1993): 68–72.

[53]A. Wilcox, L. Kobayashi, and I. Murray, "Twenty-five Years of Obstetric Patient Satisfaction in North America: A Review of the Literature," *Journal of Perinatal and Neonatal Nursing* 10 (March 1997): 361–378; Brigitte Jordan, *Birth in Four Cultures*, 4th ed. (Prospect Heights, IL: Waveland Press, 1993); Robbie Davis-Floyd, *Birth as an American Rite of Passage* (University of California Press, 2004); Jessica Mitford, *The American Way of Birth* (Plume Pub, 1993).

[54]Sara Bower, "The Obstetrical Nurse," *American Journal of Nursing* 15 (June 1915): 734–735.

have become vocal in determining the kind of obstetric care they prefer,[55] but medical and hospital policies, insurance requirements, and fear of legal repercussions limit the choices available. As burgeoning technology continues to require ever-more technically proficient scientific practitioners, the problem of humanizing scientific care surfaces again and again.[56] The evidence, from outcomes research, is that nurses who would provide effective nursing care must temper needed scientific interventions with a compassionate approach that also nurtures patients' individual, human needs.

Leah Curtin, a nationally recognized nurse leader has said it well: "We need conscience to temper our technology—to add that touch which will make it strong and effective in producing human well-being. This is the trend that will—and must—dominate the future."[57] Envisioning nursing into the twenty-first century, Curtin reminds nurses:

> The humanity of the patient is at the core of the service he or she needs. Thus, the clinical care of the patient comprises only one aspect of care—and often not even the most important one. The professional relationship's very foundation is the mutual humanity of its participants.[58]

Today's expectant parents continue to need competent nurses who know how to give the best of scientific care by developing relationships that recognize and support the individual needs of patients, with or without their carefully conceived birth plans.

Historical evidence is powerful. The record shows that nurses' energies in the early years of the profession were used to meet the expectations and requirements of medical science and its practitioners. Nurses succeeded admirably in promoting scientific birth. The question remains: Who benefited the most: the patient or the doctor?

ACKNOWLEDGMENTS

My appreciation to Springer Publishing for permission to reprint portions of article previously published in *Nursing History Review:* Sylvia Rinker, "To Cultivate a Feeling of Confidence: The Nursing of Obstetric Patients, 1890–1940," *Nursing History Review* 8 (2000): 117–142.

---

[55]An ever-growing number of websites offer support and information by and for pregnant women who are seeking to have a say in their birth experiences. Just a few examples are: http://www.earthmother.org, http://www.birthmattersva.org, http://www.ican-online.org, http://www.safebirthohio.org.

[56]Linda Kobert, "Are Universal Precautions Changing the 'Nurture' of Obstetric Nursing?" *American Journal of Nursing* 89 (December 1989): 1609.

[57]Leah Curtin was editor-in-chief of the journal *Nursing Management* for 20 years and is a frequent speaker on nursing trends and leadership. Leah Curtin, *Nursing Into the 21st Century* (Springhouse, PA: Springhouse Corporation, 1996), 62.

[58]Curtin, *Nursing Into the 21st Century,* 41.

CHAPTER 9

Nursing Patients With Cancer in the 1950s: New Issues and Old Challenges

Brigid Lusk

One spring morning in 1951, student nurse Rose Marie Chioni was assigned to care for a 38-year-old woman dying of cancer. Chioni was a first-year student at a central Illinois hospital, and her new patient, whose cheerfulness and attractiveness was in stark contrast to her devastating diagnosis, deeply impressed her. The patient's cancer had announced itself the previous summer, when she began having irregular vaginal bleeding, abdominal pain, nausea, and vomiting. She lost 44 lbs over the next few months. Out of fear or ignorance or concern for costs, the young woman did not seek medical help until November of 1950. She was treated with x-rays and radium. She received whole blood and liver extract for her anemia. Now there was no more that could be done. Being responsible for a dying woman not much older than herself must have presented Chioni with an awesome nursing challenge. Sadly, at that time most patients suffering from cancer ultimately presented similar challenges as their lives came to a close. Her patient was vomiting, bleeding from the vagina, had shortness of breath, and was in pain, very weak, pale, and doubtless scared. Chioni "hoped that [she] would be able to cope with her problems, and make her last days as pleasant as possible."[1]

[1]Rose Marie Chioni Nursing Care Study, May 15, 1951. Rose Chioni Coll. box 1, folder 3, Center for Nursing Historical Inquiry, Claude Moore Health Sciences Library, University of Virginia.

Chioni wanted to have the patient sit up to help her breathe, but the woman couldn't because she was weak from loss of blood. Her patient was constantly hemorrhaging, in spite of being given koagamin to coagulate the blood and ergotrate to contract the uterus. Under Chioni's care, her patient was given whole blood and intravenous hydration. She was given injections of demerol, a narcotic, every 4 hours which "made her restful and stopped her moaning, thus relieving the family also." Chioni bathed her patient and noted her deep labored breathing, her dry skin, and her pallor, and worried about her susceptibility to pressure ulcers. She rubbed her patient's back and legs with lotion and placed warm cloths over her eyelids to moisten them because they were stuck together. The patient then "appeared much more comfortable." Chioni and the other nurses turned her patient every half hour, which frequently caused large blood clots to be expelled from the vagina. She was incontinent of urine, and a catheter was inserted. She had a "tenacious collection of dark mucous in her throat." Chioni administered mouth care and taught the family how to lubricate the patient's lips with oil. She understood that ". . . they seemed to feel better when they thought they were doing something to make her feel better." Chioni talked to the family about the common warning signs of cancer and urged them to go to their doctor at once if they experienced any of them. They assured her they would. Finally, in the early hours of the third day after admission, Chioni's patient "was breathing irregularly and her pulse was 54 and very weak. The family, doctors, and supervisor were notified." The young woman died a few minutes later.[2]

Rose Marie Chioni had been assigned to write a nursing care study on one of her patients. Because she chose this young woman with cancer, and because, after a distinguished nursing career that included the position of dean at the University of Virginia School of Nursing, Chioni archived her papers, we have an opportunity to observe in some detail one instance of the nursing care of patients with cancer at mid-century. This was a time of new treatments for cancer, but old fears of the disease persisted. This woman had received innovative radiation therapy, but she had also not sought medical help for months after she first became ill.

The question of what nurses actually do, the scope of their unique practice, can be difficult to isolate. A reflection on nurses' roles in cancer care in the 1950s, as new and complex treatments were introduced, may help nurses today express what nursing is and what nursing does. With the decline in illness

---

[2]Rose Marie Chioni Nursing Care Study, May 15, 1951. Rose Chioni Coll. box 1, folder 3, Center for Nursing Historical Inquiry, Claude Moore Health Sciences Library, University of Virginia.

arising from infectious diseases, cancer rose to become the second leading cause of death in the United States in the 1920s and has maintained this dubious distinction.[3] During the 1940s and 1950s, early diagnosis coupled with radical surgery and, perhaps, radiation, were the primary means to cure or inhibit cancer. Anticancer drugs such as nitrogen mustard, folic acid antagonists, and adrenocorticotrophic hormone were just starting to be employed.[4] But without any doubt, in spite of these medical interventions, nursing care was absolutely crucial to these patients' well-being through the course of their disease. Nursing patients with cancer called for the full range of nurses' generalist knowledge and expertise. Nurses needed to be skilled in surgical care, nutrition, hydration, and elimination care, as well as comfort measures, that included pain control and emotional support.

In the 1950s, new issues in cancer care confronted nurses. And they responded well. Nurses invented ways to help patients cope following ever-more invasive surgeries. They protected their patients and themselves from the side effects of radiation. And they followed medical orders, although highly troubling to many, by concealing a diagnosis of cancer. These topics will serve as a framework to both tease out examples of nursing practice and to illustrate the sometimes uncomfortable position that physicians and nurses found themselves in when caring for patients with cancer during these years.

NURSING CARE AND CANCER SURGERY

After experiences gained during the World War II, cancer surgery in the 1940s and 1950s explored the very limits of the human tolerance for extensive surgery. The belief was that the more tissue that could be removed, the greater the chance that all the cancerous cells would be eradicated. During these years, radical surgeries were performed for head and neck cancers; for lung, bladder, and gastric tumors; and for breast and uterine cancers. It was the age of heroics. Katherine Nelson, noted cancer nursing specialist and educator in the 1950s, recalled first hearing about a hemicorporectomy, where the patient's

---

[3]James T. Patterson, *The Dread Disease: Cancer and Modern American Culture* (Cambridge, MA: Harvard University Press, 1987), 82; "U.S. Cancer Statistics: 1999–2005 Incidence and Mortality Web Based Report," http://apps.nccd.cdc.gov/uscs/ (accessed October 15, 2009).

[4]Gordon C. Zubrod, "Historic Milestones in Curative Chemotherapy," *Seminars in Oncology* 6 (1979): 490–505.

body below the waist was amputated, from one of her students. The student seemed to be in shock. "Don't talk to me, Miss Nelson, . . . [D]on't talk to me, Miss Nelson . . . Because at Memorial Hospital this morning they cut a patient in half." Nelson herself was greatly moved and distressed.[5]

Although hemicorporectomies were extremely rare, other disfiguring surgeries that aimed to cut out all cancer cells were common. The nurses' role in the aftercare of patients following such drastic surgeries involved support in the immediate acute postoperative phase and for weeks or months afterward as the patients learned to manage their reconfigured bodies. For surgeons, the surgery itself was very often the height of their patient involvement. Jerome Urban, a renowned surgeon from the 1940s and 1950s, specialized in what he termed the "extended radical mastectomy," a radical mastectomy made even more traumatic through the additional removal of some ribs. When asked about postmastectomy care in 1948, Urban replied "Oh, I leave all that to the nurses."[6] Nurses worked with these patients to help them heal their surgical wounds and resume some semblance of normalcy. They cleansed tracheostomy tubes, inserted feeding tubes, fitted cups to ureters opening onto the abdominal wall, irrigated colostomies, and maintained pressure dressings and arm elevation following a radical mastectomy.[7]

Mastectomies

At the mid-century, nearly 70% of American women with breast cancer underwent a radical mastectomy.[8] William Halsted, a key figure in the professionalization of American surgery in the late nineteenth century, is renowned for developing this technique. Halsted reasoned that breast cancer was a local disease, growing in a systematic fashion from tissue to lymph nodes. Thus Halsted aimed to remove all trace of cancer in the breast area through removal of the breast, nearby lymph nodes, and the underlying fascia and pectoral

---

[5]"Those Were Hard Days Scripts, ONS Interview With Kay Nelson," Katherine Nelson, box 4, folder 2, Oncology Nursing Society, Pittsburgh, PA.

[6]Katherine Nelson, "The History of Cancer Nursing in the Nursing Curriculum 1860–1951," in *Cancer Nurses Make it Happen*, eds. Vera Keare and Videen McGaughey (Wallingford, CT: ACS Connecticut Division, 1987), 1–9.

[7]"Memorial Hospital Reference Book for Nurses, 1950," RG 153, box 1, folder 2, Memorial Sloan-Kettering Cancer Center, Rockefeller Archives Center.

[8]Barron H. Lerner, *The Breast Cancer Wars* (New York: Oxford University Press, 2001): 4; Alfred M. Popma, "Cancer of the Breast," *American Journal of Nursing* 57 (1957): 1570–1574.

muscles of the chest wall. A skin graft from the thigh was often needed to cover the excision.[9] Halsted's breast cancer dictums of the previous century were still followed by most U.S. surgeons until the late 1960s.

After surgery, these women had not lost only a breast. Their chest wall was deformed following loss of muscle, with a hollow area beneath the clavicle and in the axilla.[10] Most women then underwent radiation therapy and possibly either administration of male sex hormones (testosterone) or removal (sometimes radiation) of their ovaries. Some women also had their adrenal glands removed, necessitating lifelong administration of cortisol, or even their pituitary gland, requiring lifelong administration of thyroid extract and pitressin snuff.[11] About 20% of patients developed elephantiasis (immense, firm, swelling) of the affected arm due to lymphatic blockage.[12] "Radical surgery," New York nurse Clara Walter wrote in 1956, caused "untold suffering and human degradation. I see patients brutally tortured everyday [sic]—though the torture is inflicted with the most humane intentions."[13] Another nurse, Genevieve Waples Smith, wrote: "I have heard doctors tell medical and nursing students what a mutilating operation a radical mastectomy is—but with never a suggestion as to how they might make it seem less traumatic."[14] Indeed, some physicians advised radical mastectomy patients to "Put an old stocking in their bra and get on with their lives,"[15]

Virginia Dericks, an operating room supervisor and nursing instructor at Cornell University New York Hospital, set about to improve patient care following a mastectomy. Forming a nursing committee, Dericks and her nurses identified particularly difficult times for the patients, such as when the dressing was first changed, when the patient first looked at her wound, or when the patient first looked in a mirror.[16] Her committee found that "falsies," bra

---

[9]Lerner, 20–21.
[10]Lerner, 32–33.
[11]"Doctors' Lecture Notes, Breast Tumors, 1956, 1957," Virginia Dericks Papers, box 1, folder 6, Center for Nursing Historical Inquiry, Claude Moore Health Sciences Library, Historical Collections, University of Virginia.
[12]"Doctors' Lecture Notes, Breast Tumors, 1948," Virginia Dericks Papers, box 1, folder 6, Center for Nursing Historical Inquiry, Claude Moore Health Sciences Library, Historical Collections, University of Virginia.
[13]Quoted in Lerner, pp. 105–106.
[14]Genevieve Waples Smith, "When a Breast Must Be Removed," *American Journal of Nursing* 50 (1950): 335–336, 336.
[15]Lerner, 142.
[16]"Notes for Teaching, 1954–1966," Virginia Dericks Papers, box 2, folder 14, Center for Nursing Historical Inquiry, Claude Moore Health Sciences Library, Historical Collections, University of Virginia.

inserts worn to increase appearance of breast size, were less traumatic to see and try on than an actual prosthesis. Nurses were advised to compliment patients on how they looked when dressed and ready to go home. Breast prostheses were introduced gradually—either by the hospital or outpatient department nurse. As part of their work, Dericks and her committee members interviewed salespeople from 35 New York area shops that sold breast prostheses. They found several different types—four of sponge rubber, one air filled, and one filled with fluid. The most popular was a fluid-filled one, but Dericks liked the sponge rubber prostheses the best because the form was individually molded to the contours of the woman's chest wall "and extended up to the axilla, filling in the hollow which exists in so many cases."[17] In 1955, Dericks reported on an interview she had had with a nurse in a physician's office who met with postmastectomy patients to help them adjust to postoperative life. While this nurse met with women following their mastectomy, the patients' husbands met with the doctor to discuss "some of the psychological factors involved since the attitude of a married woman with a breast removed seems so dependent on her husband's acceptance and understanding of her."[18]

Colostomies

Colostomies, commonly constructed to bypass a cancerous growth, presented a devastating affront to the patient's self-image as well as significant management problems for affected patients in the 1950s. In this preplastic and predisposable era, and as colostomy appliances were developed and improved, nurses of the 1940s and 1950s experimented with bags and dressings. They tried ways to eliminate odor, and used various ointments and pastes to protect the skin.[19]

Nurses were also deeply involved with helping these patients manage the difficult procedures associated with colostomy care. Following daily irrigation, nurses helped their patients apply a bandage to cover the stoma for the rest of the day. Some patients were inventive—one had a friend make her a

---

[17]"Mastectomy Patients Studied—1954–1962," Virginia Dericks Papers, box 2, folder 15, Center for Nursing Historical Inquiry, Claude Moore Health Sciences Library, Historical Collections, University of Virginia.

[18]"Mastectomy Patients Studied, Minutes January 12, 1955," Virginia Dericks Papers, box 2, folder 15, Center for Nursing Historical Inquiry, Claude Moore Health Sciences Library, Historical Collections, University of Virginia.

[19]"Colostomy Care, Minutes of the Meeting of the New York Hospital Committee on Care of Colostomy patients, 1947–1957," Virginia Dericks papers, box 1, folder 10, Center for Nursing Historical Inquiry Collection, Claude Moore Health Sciences Library, Historical Collections, University of Virginia.

belt with a pouch, held around her stomach with hooks and eyes. Whenever necessary, a fresh piece of material was inserted into this pouch.[20] Others placed dressings or rags over the opening and held them in place with a long piece of cloth tied around the waist. Not surprisingly, when Virginia Dericks discussed colostomy patients with her students she told them that, above all, they must "stick with the patient." The most important traits in dealing with colostomy patients, Dericks wrote in her lecture notes, were "sympathy and understanding, knowledge, skill with procedures, and perseverance with solving problems."[21]

There were indeed problems, many of which were associated with irrigating the bowel through the colostomy—a mainstay of colostomy care during the 1950s. Initially the nurse, then the patient when she or he was able, inserted a tube into the stoma and irrigated it with water until the fluid returned clear. Effectively managing this procedure was a significant postoperative achievement. When one patient succeeded in doing her irrigation unaided for the first time, she recalled having her doctor, the head nurse, and the student nurse all come in to congratulate her.[22] Other nurses were less supportive. The following patient's story is quoted at length because it illustrates how essential good nursing care was and just how devastating inadequate nursing could be. This patient suffered from rectal cancer with extensive metastasis and had transferred to the local convalescent hospital from an acute care facility.

> Had an awful time there at first. Had diarrhea, bed would be "soakin" in the morning. Was irrigating lge. (sic) bowel with 10 cans a day. One nurse up there told me "we don't help people up here." Said I would have to do it myself. I didn't know where the bathroom was or what the set-up was. I didn't irrigate for three days, and "it was awful." Then that nurse was "Off" and a nice little one was on. She took me up to the room, had a hook put up for me where I could reach it to put my own water in the can, she cut the tube off for me so it would fit better, and everything went fine. I could put the water in without standing up. Then a nurse from "Memorial" came up. . . . She helped me most by talking. I was scared, she explained to me about the operation and the "healing process." She suggested that I take Sitz baths for

[20]"Colostomy Care Patient Interviews, 1951," Virginia Dericks Papers, box 1, folder 11, Center for Nursing Historical Inquiry, Claude Moore Health Sciences Library, Historical Collections, University of Virginia.

[21]"Introduction to Surgical Nursing, 1959," Virginia Dericks Papers, box 1, folder 7, Center for Nursing Historical Inquiry, Claude Moore Health Sciences Library, Historical Collections, University of Virginia.

[22]"Colostomy Care Patient Interviews, 1951," Virginia Dericks Papers, box 1, folder 11, Center for Nursing Historical Inquiry, Claude Moore Health Sciences Library, Historical Collections, University of Virginia.

> the mucus. It helps some. She helped me a lot, and told me that if I ever had any questions I could call and find out the answers.[23]

Many patients with colostomies also had a perineal wound, where the cancer had been excised from the rectum, which presented another troublesome area for the patient and nurse. Again the following example, taken from Dericks' records, illustrates good nursing care. A patient complained that he had been coming to the clinic for months complaining of a constant seepage of mucus from this site. Some doctors told him to take a sitz bath while others told him not to. He had avoided soap because he thought he was supposed to. After 8 months, he talked with an "older nurse" who told him to keep it clean with lots of soap and water. This treatment was successful.[24]

Specialized nursing care was needed for many other types of cancer operations, as surgeons invented new ways to cut out growths while maintaining essential bodily functions through fashioning new openings or connections. As with nursing care for patients following mastectomies and colostomies, nurses played a key role in helping these patients adjust to, and live with, their altered bodies.

NURSING CARE AND RADIATION

Radiation was the other major tool available at mid-century to eradicate or inhibit cancer. During the Cold War era of the 1950s, nuclear radiation for cancer treatments generated intense scientific interest, resulting in the development of high-voltage machines and the use of radioactive isotopes.[25] By the end of the decade, radioactive isotopes such as cobalt 60, gold 198, iodine 131, and phosphorus 32 were in use but were considered primarily palliative rather than curative.[26] Most patients with cancer in the 1940s and 1950s were

---

[23]"Colostomy Care Patient Interviews, 1951," Virginia Dericks Papers, box 1, folder 11, Center for Nursing Historical Inquiry, Claude Moore Health Sciences Library, Historical Collections, University of Virginia.

[24]"Colostomy Care Patient Interviews, 1951," Virginia Dericks Papers, box 1, folder 11, Center for Nursing Historical Inquiry, Claude Moore Health Sciences Library, Historical Collections, University of Virginia.

[25]Ellen Leopold, *Under the Radar: Cancer and the Cold War* (New Brunswick, NJ: Rutgers University Press, 2009).

[26]Renilda Hilkemeyer, "Nursing Care of Cancer Patients in Hospital and Home," *CA-Bulletin of Cancer Progress* 8 (July–August 1958): 122–125, 128–129; Benedict J. Duffy, "Atomic Energy in the Diagnosis and Treatment of Malignant Diseases," *American Journal of Nursing* 55 (1955): 434–437.

treated by one of the more traditional radiation sources, x-rays, radium, or radon, usually in addition to surgical removal of the tumor.

The effects of radiation therapy frequently caused increased suffering to these patients who were already traumatized by the disease itself. Patients, particularly those who had had abdominal radiation, experienced nausea and vomiting, they had no appetite, and they suffered from general malaise.[27] After about 10 days of radiation, the skin became reddened, sore, and blisters sometimes appeared. A few days later, the area became moist and the skin started to slough off. The patient experienced intense tenderness and pain in the area. Nurses were warned to always call this an area of erythema (the medical term or euphemism for redness) and not a burn. The word burn had negative connotations and might suggest that a mistake had been made.[28]

No food was given for 2 to 3 hours following x-ray therapy, but nurses encouraged their patients to drink refreshing fluids such as citrus juices, sour wine, or ginger ale.[29] Blisters were sometimes opened on the damaged skin to properly cleanse the area,[30] but then nurses had to keep the area as clean as possible to avoid infection. Later, as the skin hardened, ointments such as lanolin or shortening (Crisco) were applied to keep the area from drying. Alcohol, dressings, and tape were avoided.[31]

Before the development of high-voltage x-ray machines that could reach tumors deep within the body, radium was the treatment of choice for deep-seated cancers. Radium was placed inside a cavity, such as the uterus, or inserted into the tissues of a cancerous growth. Applicators made of silver, gold, or platinum were filled with radium and then secured inside a rubber or lead tube. These applicators were fashioned with an eyelet through which a waxed thread was placed. The radium applicators

---

[27]"Surgical Nursing, 1948–1959, Radiation, Dr. Jensen 10/57" Virginia Dericks Papers, box 1, folder 6, Center for Nursing Historical Inquiry, Claude Moore Health Sciences Library, Historical Collections, University of Virginia.

[28]American Cancer Society, *A Cancer Source Book for Nurses* (New York: American Cancer Society, 1950): 39; Helen Young and Eleanor Lee, *Essentials of Nursing* (New York: G.P. Putnam's, 1948): 425–430.

[29]Margaret Hopp, "Roentgen Therapy and the Nurse," *American Journal of Nursing* 41 (1941): 431–433.

[30]Renilda Hilkemeyer, "A Glimpse into the Past of Cancer Nursing," *Dimensions in Oncology Nursing* 5 (1991): 5–8.

[31]"Surgical Nursing, 1948–1959, Radiation, Dr. Jensen 10/57" Virginia Dericks Papers, box 1, folder 6, Center for Nursing Historical Inquiry, Claude Moore Health Sciences Library, Historical Collections, University of Virginia; Hilkemeyer, "Nursing Care of Cancer Patients in Hospital and Home," 122–125, 128–129.

were then either sutured in place or held in place through taping down the waxed thread. The threads also allowed for easy withdrawal of the radium.[32]

Radium was usually the treatment of choice for patients with gynecological cancers. In Chicago's large public hospital, the Cook County Hospital, records from the gynecology ward in the late 1940s vividly reveal the widespread use of this treatment. Every month the census showed that there were 8 to 15 patients with radium implants in a ward with about 100 patients.[33] Most probably this was for cancer of the uterus. Public health nurses also came into extensive contact with cancer patients in their homes, including those who had received radiation. In reviewing the caseload of a visiting nurses' agency in 1950, nurse researcher Rosalie I. Peterson found that 3% of the patients were suffering from cancer. Of these, 82% had received some type of surgery, 28% had received x-rays, and 11% had undergone radium therapy.[34]

The inexhaustible harvesting of a dense, inert gaseous radionuclide from radium, known as radon, gave many more cancer sufferers access to radiation. Radon was collected in capillary-type tubes of gold or platinum. Sometimes it was clipped into tiny pieces, forming what were known as "radon seeds." Behind a lead shield and using sterile technique, nurses placed these radon seeds into the tips of interstitial needles. These radon seeds were then implanted into cancerous growths.[35]

Nursing care for patients with radium implants was complex and demanded extensive skills along with appreciation for the dangerous substance itself, as these patients emitted radiation while the radium was in place. Typical nursing care included providing nourishing food, maintaining a patient on bed rest, administering codeine for pain, encouraging fluids in order to dilute the toxins, and watching the skin for redness. Radium implants in the uterus required frequent douches, as the discharge of necrotic tissue might be profuse. After the douche, a tight perineal pad was applied so that the radium stayed in place if the patient retched or vomited. These

---

[32]Richard F. Mould, *A Century of X-Rays and Radioactivity in Medicine* (Bristol, Avon, Philadelphia: Institute of Physics Publishing), 1993.

[33]"Cook County Hospital School of Nursing Annual Report 1944," Cook County Hospital, box 13A, folder 233, Health Sciences Library, Special Collections, University of Illinois at Chicago.

[34]Rosalie I. Peterson, "An Analysis of the Cancer Caseload of the Nonofficial Nursing Agency Rendering Bedside Nursing Service in the Home in a Large Metropolitan City. Dissertation, 1950," box 3, folder 20, Oncology Nursing Society, Pittsburgh, PA.

[35]Max Cutler, "The Radium Treatment of Cancer. Parts 1 and 2," *American Journal of Nursing* 34 (1934): 641–648, 763–767; Katherine Nelson, "What is Radiation Medicine?" *Nursing World* 133, no. 4 (1959): 18–21, 33.

patients were routinely catheterized because the tight packing made it difficult for them to pass urine.[36] Patients with radium implants in their mouths needed frequent mouth irrigations to flush out dead tissue; they were unable to talk and received a liquid diet by sucking through glass tubes. Patients with radium needles inserted into the breast needed to remain quietly in bed with their arm held up on a pillow or in a sling. Those with radium in the rectum were placed on a rubber ring and given tincture of opium to constipate and avert bowel movements during the therapy.[37]

Radium was tremendously expensive as well as dangerous, and nurses had to make sure it was not accidently lost in a bedpan or among the sheets. Only nurses (and some hospitals required a second nurse to act as a witness) emptied these patients' bedpans. At Memorial Hospital in New York, nurses stopped everything if a radium applicator was missing. The water was turned off, no toilets were flushed, no laundry was disposed of, and no one was allowed in or out of the area until the radium was located.[38] Nurses picked up radium that became dislodged using long-handled forceps and then quickly placed the radium-loaded applicator into the bedside lead container.[39] The radium was removed at the scheduled end of treatment. While the physician actually removed the radium in its applicator, the nurses removed the wax threads attached to it. The nurse then washed the radium applicator in peroxide, followed by ether and then alcohol before replacing it in the lead container.[40]

Patients with radium implanted were constantly emitting radiation and therefore posed a danger to those in their immediate area. Contacts with others—visitors and healthcare staff—were restricted.[41] Nurse educator Katherine Nelson advised nurses that they should plan their care so that they kept their contact with an irradiated patient to a minimum. She told nurses that a conversation held from the doorway could be just as beneficial as one standing by the bedside.[42] Nurses working extensively with radiation sources were usually monitored by film badges.[43]

---

[36]Fay Thomas, "Surgery and Gynecology, Notebooks, 1944," Thomas Vaden Collection, box 2, Claude Moore Health Sciences Library, Historical Collections, University of Virginia.
[37]Nelliana Best, "Radiotherapy and the Nurse," *American Journal of Nursing* 50 (1950): 140–143.
[38]"Memorial Hospital Reference Book for Nurses, 1950," RG 153, box 1, folder 2, Memorial Sloan-Kettering Cancer Center, Rockefeller Archives Center.
[39]Young and Lee, 425–430; Nelson, "What is Radiation Medicine?" 18–21, 33.
[40]Young and Lee, 425–430.
[41]Hilkemeyer, "Nursing Care of Cancer Patients in Hospital and Home," 122–125, 128–129.
[42]Nelson, What Is Radiation Medicine? 18–21, 33.
[43]"Memorial Hospital Reference Book for Nurses, 1950," RG 153, box 1, folder 2, Memorial Sloan-Kettering Cancer Center, Rockefeller Archives Center.

Concern about physician and nurse safety was not consistently apparent in the early years of the century.[44] Yet even in 1959, Katherine Nelson raised the concern that nurses were in danger from radiation. She advised nurses to decide for themselves how long they could be with patients and to not rely on doctors telling them that they would be safe. "I know of instances," she wrote "where nurses were told by doctors: "Oh, don't worry about radiation, it won't hurt you."[45] Yet there is little evidence that nurses had the knowledge necessary to protect themselves as they cared for these patients. Recalling these years, cancer nursing authority Renilda Hilkemeyer said that nurses' knowledge in this area was "practically nil."[46] There were few sources where nurses could have learned about radiation and nursing care. A review of nursing textbooks found only one that addressed radiation therapies in any depth, and that content was limited to a few pages.[47] Physicians taught nursing students about radiation therapies, but lecture notes did not address nurses' safety. Hilkemeyer wrote that her 1967 article on nursing care in radium therapy was widely distributed by the American Cancer Society because there was so little information available for nurses at that time.[48]

Some nurses, concerned about the danger, refused to take care of patients undergoing treatment with radium or radioactive isotopes.[49] Their refusal was couched in the political issues of the period; the Cold War and the perceived threat of nuclear annihilation, nuclear testing, and its resultant contamination all contributed to the public's fear of radiation at the time. Awareness of nurses' limited knowledge of therapeutic radiation coupled with the typical physician's inexperience in the field, further explains their position.

A CANCER DIAGNOSIS IN THE 1950s

Rose Marie Chioni's patient was in the last stages of her disease. She must have known that she was dying of cancer even if no one had actually told her. Typically, patients during this time were not told they had cancer; they were

---

[44]Brigid Lusk, "Prelude to specialization: U.S. Cancer Nursing, 1920–1950," *Nursing Inquiry* 12 (2005): 269–277.

[45]Nelson, "What Is Radiation Medicine?" 18–21, 33.

[46]Hilkemeyer, "A Glimpse into the Past of Cancer Nursing," 5–8, 7.

[47]Young and Lee, 425–430. The few paragraphs related to x-rays and radium/radon in the fourth edition of Bertha Harmer and Virginia Henderson's *Textbook of Principles and Practice of Nursing* (New York: Macmillan, 1948) do not address nurses' safety.

[48]Hilkemeyer, "A Glimpse into the Past of Cancer Nursing," 5–8, 7.

[49]Nelson, *Nursing World,* 18–21, 33.

left to come to that realization by themselves. Physicians in the United States during the 1950s were at the peak of their paternalistic professional authority and power.[50] They invariably ordered that a diagnosis of cancer should be hidden from those who were most intimately affected—the patients themselves. The practice of keeping a distressing diagnosis such as cancer hidden from the patient had been standard practice for decades. It was commonly considered to be humane, to foster a necessary sense of hope, and to facilitate patients' compliance in the proposed treatment.[51] However, concealing the diagnosis placed nurses in a particularly awkward position as nurses, unlike doctors, had extensive personal contact with their patients. As nurses helped patients irrigate their colostomies or dressed their surgical incisions, they could not reveal the truth. Patients were left to suspect that they might have cancer and nurses were left wondering what patients knew.[52]

This tension came through in a series of home interviews carried out in the late 1940s under the direction of an anthropologist.[53] He was interested in how people coped with colostomies at home. Virginia Dericks, then chair of the colostomy committee at Cornell University New York Hospital, provided him with the names of some of her recently discharged patients.[54] In addition to information about colostomy management, these interviews revealed the patients' fears of cancer and their suspicion that they probably had the disease. One woman, with a recurrence of her cancer, talked about her hope that her pain was due to some indigestible okra she had eaten, but confessed that she was worried that it was really cancer. She had been told she was "fine." Sometimes patients were told that they had another problem or were given

---

[50]Leopold, 3, 211–212. Couched in the debate over informed consent, Leopold discussed the unquestioned authority of physicians over patients, particularly women with cancer, in the 1950s. Also see Paul Starr, *Social Transformation of American Medicine* (New York: Basic Books, 1982): 389–391. Starr describes the increasing distrust of medical authority by members of the women's movement in the 1970s.

[51]Eleanor E. Cockerill, "The Cancer Patient as a Person," *Public Health Nursing* 40 (February 1948): 78–83.

[52]"Mastectomy Patients Studied, 1954–1962," Virginia Dericks Papers, box 2, folder 15, Center for Nursing Historical Inquiry, Claude Moore Health Sciences Library, Historical Collections, University of Virginia.

[53]"Colostomy Care Patient Interviews, 1951," Virginia Dericks Papers, box 1, folder 11, Center for Nursing Historical Inquiry, Claude Moore Health Sciences Library, Historical Collections, University of Virginia. Dericks recalled that the researcher was an anthropologist who had given these records to her when he left the university. Personal communication with the author, November 2003.

[54]"Colostomy Care Patient Interviews, 1951," Virginia Dericks Papers, box 1, folder 11, Center for Nursing Historical Inquiry, Claude Moore Health Sciences Library, Historical Collections, University of Virginia.

no information at all. One patient, with cancer of the rectum and extensive metastasis, was told she had colitis. Another patient, after being reassured by her doctor that there was nothing wrong with her, had overheard this same physician tell her husband that she was "a very sick woman but she doesn't know it." When her husband and her sister returned from meeting with the doctor, they told her that she had an infection and "needed a lot of rest." A middle-aged woman confided: "A couple of times they said, 'Oh, you'll live to be eighty,' and things like that." Actually, this denial of her illness by the hospital staff convinced the woman, correctly, that she had cancer.[55]

The physicians' near-complete authority and their paternalistic attitudes regarding what patients should be told are epitomized in some 1948 notes of a doctor's lectures to student nurses. This surgeon told his patients suffering from breast cancer that they had a "tumor" that must be removed in case it turned into cancer. If, however, a patient refused the surgery she was essentially punished for her boldness. In the presence of her family, she was told that she had cancer and that she would die of it unless she allowed the surgeon to operate.[56]

Katherine Nelson was concerned and angered by this practice of deception. She described patients who would go to surgery and return with a colostomy. As she wrote, this was "devastating for the patient . . . they would turn on the nurses, and they would fight us, they would, you know, they'd scream at us. And they'd say, 'What did you do to me?' So we were caught between our loyalty and ethical responsibility to the medical profession and the fact that they weren't telling the patients and the patients were coming to us."[57] Nelson was once asked by a nursing supervisor to visit a postmastectomy patient because the nurses were worried about her. The patient told Nelson that she was so relieved that her cancer was removed. "The doctor tells me it's all gone, it's all out," she said. She told Nelson that she could face death, but she was a single mother and if she was dying she would have to make arrangements for her children. Now she did not have to worry. Nelson went to look at her chart.

---

[55]"Colostomy Care Patient Interviews, 1951," Virginia Dericks Papers, box 1, folder 11, Center for Nursing Historical Inquiry, Claude Moore Health Sciences Library, Historical Collections, University of Virginia.

[56]"Doctors' Lecture Notes, Breast Tumors, 1948," Virginia Dericks Papers, box 1, folder 6, Center for Nursing Historical Inquiry, Claude Moore Health Sciences Library, Historical Collections, University of Virginia.

[57]"Those Were Hard Days, Scripts," Katherine Nelson, box 4, Oncology Nursing Society, Pittsburgh, PA.

The woman was, in Nelson's words, "loaded with cancer."[58] Nelson found out that this particular surgeon "opens them up, he finds a lot of cancer, he rips off the gloves and says to the interns 'close her up, close her up.' Then he lies to the patient and the nurses are left in the middle."[59] Later, Nelson reminisced that this truly put nurses "behind the eight ball."[60]

CONCLUSIONS

This review of cancer nursing from over 60 years ago gives some idea of the breadth and responsibilities of this type of nursing care. As the nursing care of cancer patients became more technical and specialized, nurses were faced with the aftermath of their patients' life-altering surgeries and had to create new ways to care for them. Many nurses rose to this challenge, and this chapter has documented their original ideas and their compassion for their patients. They demonstrated nurses' independent roles in the care of post-surgical cancer patients. For patients undergoing radiation, both patients and nurses relied upon scientific knowledge, the physics of radiation, to ensure that appropriate care was given and safety was maintained. Some did not do so. The nursing procedures associated with radiation administration were complex, frightening, and fraught with issues of too little information or education.

During the period studied, as cancer was more readily detected and potentially more effective treatments were developed, the issue of concealment of a cancer diagnosis is worthy of reflection. This was a common practice, repeated throughout the various sources consulted, yet was very disturbing to some nurses of the period. Inherent in the concealment was fear of the patient's reaction to the devastating news of a diagnosis of cancer. For many people, being told that they had cancer was the same as being told that they would die.

For these patients, good nursing care would become absolutely key as they recovered or as their disease progressed. And there were rewards in giving this type of nursing. To end with the care study by Rose Marie Chioni:

---

[58]"Those Were Hard Days Scripts, ONS Interview With Kay Nelson," Katherine Nelson, box 4, folder 2, Oncology Nursing Society, Pittsburgh, PA.
[59]"Those Were Hard Days Scripts, ONS Interview With Kay Nelson," Katherine Nelson, box 4, folder 2, Oncology Nursing Society, Pittsburgh, PA.
[60]"Those Were Hard Days Scripts, ONS Interview With Kay Nelson," Katherine Nelson, box 4, folder 2, Oncology Nursing Society, Pittsburgh, PA.

". . . after PM care on the last day of her life, she opened her eyes, grasped my hand, and smiled. She immediately went into a deep sleep . . . that last smile has made an impact on my mind."[61]

ACKNOWLEDGMENTS

This work was partially supported by grants from the Center for Nursing Historical Inquiry at the University of Virginia School of Nursing, the Oncology Nursing Society, and the Rockefeller Archive Center. I greatly appreciate their generous support.

---

[61]Rose Marie Chioni Nursing Care Study, May 15, 1951. Rose Chioni Coll. box 1, folder 3, Center for Nursing Historical Inquiry, Claude Moore Health Sciences Library, University of Virginia.

CHAPTER 10

Trial and Negotiation in a Technological System: Case Study of the Swan-Ganz Catheter

Kathleen G. Burke

INTRODUCTION

Healthcare is, and remains, one of the most pressing challenges facing our nation (and the world) in the twenty-first century. Almost any discussion related to improving healthcare, whether it implicates reducing costs or improving patient safety, quality, and satisfaction, usually has technology as a core component. Understanding how healthcare providers work with technology in this complex system is key to safe, effective care of patients.[1]

Nurses are the primary users of the technology in healthcare. Technology can be compelling, exciting, and demanding of nurses' time and skill.[2] Nurses, through their 24-hour presences at the patient's bedside, their creativity, comfort in taking risk with new skills, expertise, and knowledge, make the use of technology at the bedside care of the patient possible.[3] Although recent nursing literature has begun to address the relationship between

[1]Coy Smith, "New Technology Continues to Invade Healthcare: What Are the Strategic Implications/Outcomes?" *Nursing Administration Quarterly* 28, no. 2 (April/May/June 2004): 92–98.
[2]Julie A. Fairman "Alternative Visions: The Nurse—Technology Relationship in the Context of the History of Nursing," *Nursing History Review* 6 (1998): 130.
[3]Ibid., 137.

nursing and technology, there is still much we can learn from the work of nurses in this technological system. Indeed, nurses have more power over the technological system than is usually acknowledged in the literature.[4] Nurses make assessments and gather data daily to frame their decisions about what technology to use, with what patients should they use it, and when and how to use it. In many cases, if nurses do not believe the technology will help their patients, or if they do not trust the technology, or if they do not understand how to use the technology, then the technology may, according to Julie A. Fairman, "fall into disuse or fall prey to sabotage by the nurses."[5]

This chapter examines the role of nurses in the developing complex technological system of the Intensive Care Units (ICUs) during the 1970s. The introduction and early use of the Swan-Ganz catheter in the Surgical ICU (SICU) at the Hospital of University of Pennsylvania (HUP), a university-based teaching hospital in Philadelphia, Pennsylvania, serves as an exemplar illustrating the role of nurses and the decisions that they made in the use of this technology during the explosive growth of ICUs. Through the story of the early use of the Swan-Ganz catheter, we gain insight into the factors that influence the adoption of new technology in the bedside care of patients and the practice decisions nurses make as they continuously adopt new technology into the ever-changing and increasing complex practice environment.[6]

THE SURGICAL INTENSIVE CARE UNIT

Bedside practice in the ICUs during the 1970s was a dynamic time. During the late 1960s and early 1970s, many hospitals created new specialized ICUs complete with all the latest technology. The ICUs of the 1970s transformed into complex technological systems and the role of intensive care nurses, as the only constant at the patient's bedside and with their growing technical expertise and minute-to-minute patient knowledge,

---

[4]Ibid., 137.

[5]Ibid., 137.

[6]Antonella Surbone, Thomas H. Gallagher, Katherine Russell Rich, and Michael Rowe, "To Err Is Human 5 Years Later" *Journal of American Medical Association* 294, no. 14 (2005): 1758; Patricia R. Ebright et al. "Understanding the Complexity of Registered Nurse Work in Acute Care Settings," *Journal of Nursing Administration* 33, no. 12 (December 2003): 630–638.

expanded their focus beyond the "watchful vigilance" of the 1950s and the "technical/survival" care of the 1960s to become the "orchestrators of care" during the 1970s.[7]

In the fall of 1968, HUP opened a new open ward 13-bed SICU on 5 White (12 beds and one isolation room) equipped with all the state-of-the-art technology.[8] The SICU admitted three main types of patients: cardiothoracic surgical patients (CT); general surgical patients, including those who had had major abdominal surgery; and renal transplants and neurosurgical patients, including some trauma patients. The CT service was by far the most powerful service in the unit because, like many university teaching hospitals, HUP surgeons performed Coronary Artery Bypass Grafting (CABG) surgery (attachment of a saphenous vein graft to the ascending aorta to a coronary artery to bypass an occlusion) in addition to valvular (mitral and aortic) replacement surgery.[9] The rapid growth of CABG surgery in the treatment of coronary artery disease reflected the national enthusiasm for this new procedure. Coronary artery disease was causing the death of more than 600,000 people each year and incapacitating another 3.5 to 5.0 million people.[10]

The nursing staff in the SICU was young, inexperienced, bright, and enthusiastic. Most of those working there had been recruited from other medical–surgical floors in the hospital. Nurses wanted to work in the SICU because it was considered a prestigious and exciting place to work at that time. One nurse remembered, "The ICUs were considered a great place to

---

[7]Joan E. Lynaugh and Barbara L. Brush, *American Nursing From Hospital to Health System* (Cambridge, MA: Milbank Memorial Fund and Blackwell Publishers, 1996), 35–37. See also for a discussion of the early development of ICUs and the SICU at the HUP, Julie A. Fairman, "New Hospitals, New Nurses, New Spaces: The Development of Intensive Care Units, 1950–1965" (PhD, University of Pennsylvania, 1992), Chapter 5. See for a description of the role of the ICU nurse in the 1950s–1960s, Julie A. Fairman, "Watchful Vigilance: Nursing Care, Technology, and the Development of Intensive Care Units," *Nursing Research* 41(January–February, 1992): 56. Julie A. Fairman and Joan E. Lynaugh, *Critical Care Nursing: A History* (Philadelphia, PA: University of Pennsylvania Press, 1998). Kathleen G. Burke, "From Research Lab to Routine Procedure: A Case Study of the Swan-Ganz Catheter 1965–1980" (PhD, University of Pennsylvania, 2001).
[8]Paula E. Crawford, Larry W. Stephenson, Horace MacVaugh, Alden H. Harken, and L. Henry Edmunds Jr., "Is an Intermediate Cardiac Surgical Intensive Care Unit Really Necessary?" *Heart and Lung* 8 (July–August 1979): 686.
[9]Hospital of the University of Pennsylvania, Dr. Henry Edmunds Records, Cardiothoracic Surgery 1956–1990.
[10]David S. Jones, "Visions of Cure Visualization, Clinical Trials and Controversies in Cardiac Therapeutics, 1968–1998," *ISIS* 91 (2000): 504–541. W. Stan Wilson "Aortocoronary Bypass Surgery II: An Updated Review," *Heart and Lung* 3 (May–June 1974): 435–453.

work and it was an honor to be asked to work in them because 'only the best nurses worked in the ICUs.'"[11] They were also ambitious; many of the nurses came to HUP to obtain their bachelor's or master's degrees in nursing from the University of Pennsylvania [Penn].[12] Louise Riley, for example, came to HUP in 1973, with a bachelor's degree from Villanova University in Pennsylvania and with plans to obtain her master's degree in nursing from Penn. Riley first worked on a medical–surgical floor at HUP before she was recruited to work in the SICU in 1973. Riley described what it was like in the SICU at that time:

> [It was] overwhelming. When I was in nursing school [Villanova] we didn't have our own hospital and we mostly went to small community hospitals and I think I did one or two days in an ICU there. When I went to the SICU, I didn't even know there were such things as a-lines [systemic arterial lines to measure blood pressure]. So it was a whole new world.[13]

The SICU in the 1970s was a very busy place to work. The postoperative care of CABG patients was exciting and challenging. Still, the physicians and nurses working in the unit during these times sometimes seemed overwhelmed with all the work, new technology, and responsibilities.[14] In this increasingly complex technological system, the introduction of the Swan-Ganz catheter initially slipped into use in the SICU with very little fanfare.

INTRODUCTION OF THE SWAN-GANZ CATHETER

The introduction of the Swan-Ganz catheter in patients in the SICU, although significant, was just one more new technology. Nurse Marla Broughton remembered, "There was a constant stream of things that started in the operating room (OR) and then came to the SICU with patients. The Swan-Ganz

---

[11]Patricia Naji, RN, interview, February 10, 2000, Hospital of the University of Pennsylvania.
[12]Julie A. Fairman, RN, interview, January 14, 2000, School of Nursing, University of Pennsylvania.
[13]Louise Riley, RN, interview, November 22, 1999, School of Nursing, University of Pennsylvania.
[14]Marla Broughton, RN, interview, December 14, 1999, Hospital of the University of Pennsylvania.

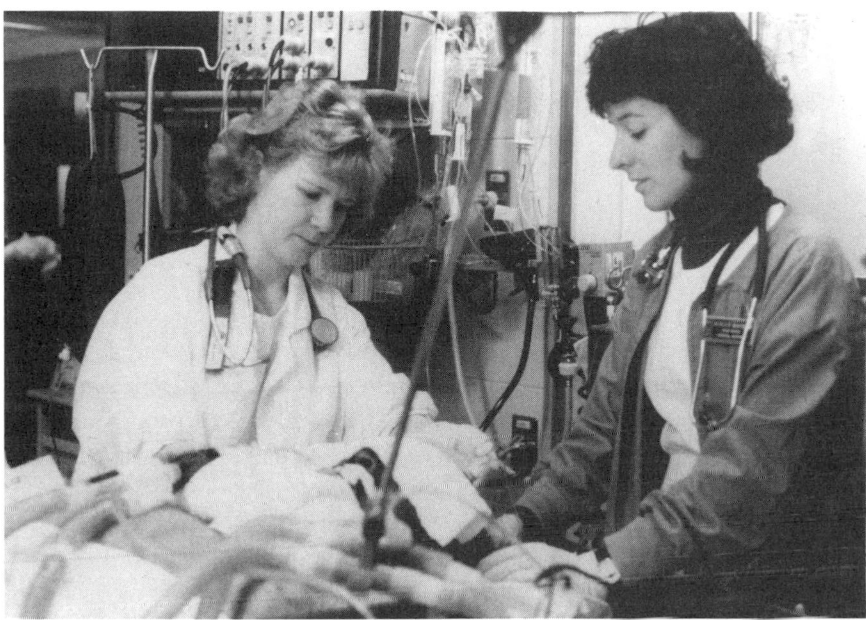

FIGURE 10.1 Hospital of the University of Pennsylvania Surgical Intensive Care Unit nurses caring for a patient, ca. late 1970/early 1980. *Reprinted with permission of The Barbara Bates Center for the Study of the History of Nursing (Philadelphia, PA).*

was probably a more significant one looking back at it."[15] According to most accounts, anesthesiologists initiated the use of the Swan-Ganz catheter in patients with the support of surgeons. Although it is not clear exactly when the introduction of the Swan-Ganz catheter in the SICU occurred, it is clear that it happened gradually and without planning. Skip Ellison, an anesthesiologist and one of the early adopters of the Swan-Ganz catheter, recalled:

> I had gone out to the Cleveland Clinic as a visiting professor sometime in the early seventies, around 1972–1973, to give a lecture on homeostasis

[15]Ibid.; H. J. C. Swan, William Ganz, James Forrester, Harold Marcus, George Diamond, and David Chonette, "Catheterization of the Heart in Man with Use of a Flow-Directed Balloon-Tipped Catheter," *The New England Journal of Medicine* 283, no. 9 (August 27, 1970): 447–451. The Swan-Ganz catheter or Pulmonary Artery Catheter (PAC) was a multilumen, radiopaque, balloon-tipped, polyvinyl chloride catheter that allowed for fast, reliable passage into the pulmonary artery at the patient's bedside for the first time. The double-lumen catheter allows for monitoring the pulmonary artery pressure and the pulmonary capillary wedge pressure (PCWP). The smallest lumen is used for balloon inflation and deflation, while the larger lumen is necessary to maintain catheter patency and to connect the catheter to a transducer and a monitor.

> and when I went there, that was where the first one [Swan-Ganz catheter] that I ever put in personally [took place] . . . So, I took it [the idea of the Swan-Ganz catheter] back [to HUP] and ordered some. It was a lot easier to order things in those days. If I didn't put in the first one [Swan-Ganz catheter] in the OR, I put in one of the very first ones. I thought it was around 1973–1974.[16]

In the beginning, only open-heart surgical patients considered to be at high risk for cardiac failure had Swan-Ganz catheters as part of their care. The Swan-Ganz catheter was inserted in the OR by anesthesiologist, who used it to measure the pulmonary artery (PA) and pulmonary capillary wedge (PCWP) pressures throughout the surgery. The Swan-Ganz catheter was then removed before the patient was taken to the SICU. That did not last very long, however, and soon the patients began arriving in the SICU with the Swan-Ganz catheter still in place. Ellison recalled:

> Well, in around "74" I wanted to do this [use the Swan-Ganz catheter in the SICU] I talked to the resident I was working with that day and I took the patient up to the unit and I said something to the nurse in report, this is this, this is that, this is what you have to watch out for. I should have really been the person that should have been there at the change of shift to make sure that the next nurse got the same information [so that they didn't have to rely on] that whispering down the lane sort of thing.[17]

The nurses in the SICU were used to the "whisper down the lane"[18] way of learning about new things because that was what happened almost every day. A patient arriving from the OR with a new piece of technology was not unusual. Broughton described the scene in the SICU when a patient arrived from the OR with a Swan-Ganz catheter:

> It [the introduction a Swan-Ganz catheter] was without very much warning, so we didn't have the transducers ready. Of course, it was the usual chaos getting things together. But then the nurse would say "What do I do with this?" and the anesthesia people would say, "Well, this is what you do, this, this and this"; that is how we learned what to do.[19]

---

[16]Skip Ellison, MD, interview, Nov. 18, 1999, Hospital of the University of Pennsylvania.
[17]Ibid.
[18]Broughton, interview.
[19]Ibid.

In the beginning the work of the SICU nurses with the Swan-Ganz catheter was very basic and functional. Broughton explained:

> It was sort of very basic in the beginning. We set up the transducers and the tubing before the patient got to the unit. Once in the unit we dutifully recorded the numbers the CVP, PA mean (mean of systolic and diastolic pressure), PCWP (Pulmonary Capillary Wedge Pressure) if somebody did one and told us about it but we really didn't know what they meant. I personally wrote down everything I saw. It was just a matter of recording information that somebody else wanted. It seems that very little attention was given to the data by the residents or the attending physicians. The Swan was not considered a big wonderful revolution to nurses at first.[20]

Initially, most nurses did not know how to interpret the PA waveforms that were displayed on the monitor. As one nurse explained, "I did not know what I was looking at on the monitor. I just wrote the numbers down. We rezeroed the transducers and calibrated the monitor. I remember doing things like that."[21] At first, the nurses were not allowed to "wedge" the catheter (inflate the balloon on the end of the catheter to measure pulmonary capillary wedge pressure). Ellison explained, "I think we thought it was too dangerous for the nurses."[22] Nurse Louise Riley explained, "We were not allowed to wedge it. I can't remember back then saying 'you know it looks like it's in the ventricle' or anything like that. That came much later."[23] Eventually some nurses started wedging the catheter themselves because they felt they needed the data and did not want to wait for a physician to do it. "After a while, when we thought that the wedge pressure was important so some of us started doing them [inflating the balloon to wedge the catheter] ourselves, who had time to find a doc."[24]

The nurses found it frustrating to work with the Swan-Ganz catheter because they knew so very little about it and because there always seemed to be a problem with it. Julie A. Fairman, a nurse who began working in the SICU in 1976, explained:

> They (Swan-Ganz) were almost more trouble than they were worth at first. They never seemed to work, they never seemed accurate. We weren't sure if the balloons were intact, we never quite really believed what it was saying. Just as we were dealing with the Swan in came cardiac output technology

---

[20]Ibid.

[21]Riley, interview.

[22]Ellison, interview.

[23]Riley, interview.

[24]Patricia Naji, RN, interview, February 2, 2000, Hospital of the University of Pennsylvania.

> with ice water and we didn't believe that either but we seemed to use that to substitute what we were getting off the Swan. At one point no one at Penn really knew what it [waveform] was supposed to look like. It was a matter of looking at something and saying hum that looks about right or maybe it's stuck someplace else. It was not a science.[25]

Broughton also described her frustrations working with the Swan-Ganz catheter:

> It [the Swan] was annoying because it flopped around and the dressings would come off, the patients were diaphoretic [sweaty]. You know the dressing would come lose [sic] you would have to change it and find a way to make it stick. And then maybe some idiot comes and pulls on the catheter; the Swan is not really in the right place and you have to get someone to put in a new one.[26]

After a few months the nurses began asking, "You know this is a pain in the neck, why I am I doing this? What is this showing?"[27] According to Ellison, Joan Richards, the head nurse at that time, approached him and said, "You know, we really would like to hear something about this."[28] So Ellison and surgeon Horace McVaugh gave small classes called in-services on what the pressures meant, the waveforms, and how the catheter worked. "We gave a series of classes and I did all three shifts several times."[29]

But many nurses did not have time to leave their patients or they missed the in-services due to days off or vacations, so they had to rely on teaching each other. Fairman explained, "We taught each other basically. They tried to do in-services but you know we were staffed so precisely I guess it was really hard to get away to any kind of in-services. You know with SICU people, we thought we knew everything anyhow."[30]

BECOMING PART OF PRACTICE: LEARNING TO TRUST

Although the use of the Swan-Ganz catheter grew rapidly, the incorporation of the data from the Swan-Ganz catheter into clinical practice was a gradual process. The nurses and physicians needed to learn to work with and trust

---

[25]Fairman, interview.
[26]Broughton, interview.
[27]Ibid.
[28]Ellison, interview.
[29]Broughton, interview.
[30]Fairman, interview.

the information the Swan-Ganz catheter provided before they used it in their clinical decision making. Broughton explained:

> It [trusting the Swan] took a while, it didn't happen overnight. It took a while for people to buy into the fact that technology did make a difference. We didn't trust it. Although I think we all thought and I still think that a very sharp nurse could pick a lot of things up just as well as technology, but you have to know what you are looking for. The information from the Swan-Ganz catheter taught us what to look for.[31]

Riley described why the data from the Swan-Ganz catheter became more meaningful once she trusted it:

> This one [the Swan-Ganz catheter] turned out to be a really good tool to manage fluid volume, which was always a problem post operatively. How much fluid did a person have onboard [sic]? Did they have additional cardiac insult intraoperatively? All these things were becoming more meaningful. The numbers that were thrown around before didn't mean a whole lot. And then we began to see the correlation between those pressures and what was seen postoperatively [changes in BP, heart rate, urine output, skin color temperature] and then you could understand better what it was all about.[32]

The SICU nurses also began making choices about how and when to include the information from the Swan-Ganz catheter into their clinical decision making and this, in turn, influenced the clinical decisions of the physicians. Nurse Joanne Konick-McMahon described the process:

> My observation is that a nurse can bring across the values of a number or physical finding to physicians either in a very positive way, this as a valuable piece of information which means a lot, or downplay the pieces of information. And I think early on we tended to downplay the information [from the Swan-Ganz catheter]. I don't know that we necessarily had a choice in terms of whether the catheter was in the patient at least in that point in time. We didn't resist in terms of not putting numbers downs [sic] or not taking care of the equipment. We were ICU nurses and we liked taking care of the equipment because we were taking care of the patients and we saw this as benefiting the patient by taking care of the equipment. But, I think

---

[31]Broughton, interview; Mary Reiser, RN, telephone interview, May 11, 2000; HUP Department of Nursing Raven Head Nurse Minutes, February 27, 1968; HUP Department of Nursing Raven/White Divisions Head Nurse Minutes, April 7, 1970. Minutes discussed the addition of an arrhythmia class starting April 22, 1970.

[32]Riley, interview.

> when it came time to making clinical decisions and helping the house staff to make clinical decisions about what to do next, I think that nurses have always had the ability to point up the information or play down the information. A nurse who was not so thrilled with the pulmonary artery catheter could give a whole litany of information in terms of changes and oh by the way, the pulmonary catheter say this but who believes it anyway. Or on the other hand you could start out with that information [PA pressure data] and then give other data to support the PA readings. We painted the picture for the house staff.[33]

The nurses caring for these complex critically ill patients believed that technology was giving them information that would help their patients, as one nurse described:

> At the time it [technology] certainly seemed to help for the most part. Because, back then, when a patient went into pulmonary edema we were doing rotating tourniquets [tourniquets applied to the legs and arms to treat congestive heart failure], and then the Swan gave us a little bit more information, like, oh, we don't have to do the rotating tourniquets we could do . . . Technology gave us the sense that we were doing the best possible thing—we believed that we were doing the best possible thing for that patient. We're offering them the best possible things we can offer, or, the most possible things. Whether they were the best is yet to be seen, it depends. So we are offering him the most there is to offer and it gives us the sense of pride in how we practice and it also adds on that aspect of guiding him, the patient, through these trouble[d] waters. And, I think, a lot of what we did, and do now, is interpretation of the technology.[34]

Even though many of new technologies consumed much of the nurses' time, for the most part, nurses did not resist incorporating the technology into their care because they believed that they were part of a team that was helping to improve patient care. As nurse Patricia Naji described:

> It seems to me it was kind of accepted, as this is the latest thing, and this is what we're doing. This is how we're monitoring our patients and it is giving us the answers that we need. Were there some frustrations with equipment? Yeah. The printer not working, all that kind of stuff, you know. So, in a sense, I think nurses could be frustrated with the equipment, not the answers it was giving us, or not the opportunity of providing better patient

---

[33]Joanne Konich-McMahon, RN, interview, July 7, 1999, School of Nursing, and University of Pennsylvania.

[34]Patricia Naji, interview.

> care, if that makes sense. I think we felt like we were partners in something, you know, it was hopefully improving patient care.[35]

The physicians and nurses did work as a team and shared some work, but the nurses established their own routine with the Swan-Ganz catheter. The nurses in the SICU were responsible for the setup and troubleshooting of the equipment. Their jobs included recording the data and interpreting all the changes and trends. Physicians inserted the catheter either in the OR or at the bedside and then left the day-to-day management of the catheter to the nurse. To the physicians, the Swan-Ganz catheter was an additional tool that gave them more data to add to their medical assessments. Initially, to the nurses the Swan-Ganz catheter was just one more piece of technology that they added to their already complex patient care. But, over time, the Swan-Ganz catheter became a useful diagnostic tool for the nurse as well. By 1980, the Swan-Ganz catheter was part of routine care of postoperative open-heart surgical patients and faded into the fabric of everyday practice in the SICU.

"It Just Kind of Blended in With Everything Else and Just Appeared at the Bedside."[36]

CONCLUSION

The introduction of the Swan-Ganz catheter into clinical practice in the SICU at the HUP was not an event but rather a gradual, individual, and opportunistic process of trial and negotiation. Initially, for the nurses, the Swan-Ganz catheter was just another piece of new technology, and their work with it was basic and functional. Their lack of knowledge about the Swan-Ganz catheter also made working with it frustrating and meaningless at times. In the beginning, in fact, nurses did not use the data the Swan-Ganz catheter provided because they did not understand it. Part of the reason for this can be attributed to the way the catheter was introduced. Little time was allotted to formal education programs for nurses. In-services; informal conversations with anesthesia, surgeons, residents, and fellows; and trial and error experiences were the only sources of information the nurse received about

---

[35]Ibid.
[36]Broughton, interview.

this new technology. As they have done in the past, though, nurses learned from each other as they "whispered down the lane."[37]

Over time and through experience with the catheter, however, nurses learned to understand and trust the data and began to incorporate it into their clinical decision making. They controlled how they used the data from the "Swan" as they "painted the picture"[38] to ensure that their patient received the care they thought the patient needed. By the end of the 1970s, the Swan-Ganz catheter was starting to become a useful diagnostic tool rather than just another new catheter or access device.

As we deal with the constant influx of new, twenty-first-century technology at the patient's bedside, the story of how nurses worked with, and learned to work with, the Swan-Ganz catheter in the 1970s has significant relevance for us. Our new clinical information systems, computer chip-based clinical monitoring devices, wireless communication devices, and clinical decision support software to improve the quality and safety of patient care are only some of the new technology that nurses interact with on a daily basis.

Yet it is important to realize that nurses make the adoption of new technology into clinical practice at the bedside possible. Although physicians have the authority to choose what technology is ordered, it is the nurse who chooses how and when to use the technology and its data in clinical decision making. In addition, as we have learned in this case study, the adoption of the data from the Swan-Ganz catheter occurred after nurses and physicians learned to trust the data through trial and negotiation. As we strive to provide quality, safe patient care in this increasingly complex healthcare environment, understanding the process of adoption and use of technology in the bedside care of patients remains a major priority.

ACKNOWLEDGMENTS

The author thanks Drs. Julie A. Fairman, Patricia D'Antonio, and Joan Lynaugh for their guidance with this project.

FURTHER READINGS

Battista, Renaldo N. "Innovation and Diffusion of Health-Related Technologies." *International Journal of Technology Assessment in HealthCare* 5 (1989): 227–248.

---

[37]Ibid.

[38]Konich-McMahon, interview.

Bernard, Gordon R. et al. "Pulmonary Artery Catheterization and Clinical Outcomes, National Heart and Lung and Blood Institute and Food and Drug Administration Workshop Report." *Journal of the American Medical Association*, 283 (May, 2000): 2568.

Burns, David, Della Burns, and Martha Shively. "Critical Care Nurses Knowledge of Pulmonary Artery Catheters." *American Journal of Critical Care* 5 (January 1996): 49–53.

Dalen, James E. and Roger C. Bone. "Is It Time to Pull the Pulmonary Artery Catheter?" *Journal of the American Medical Association* 276 (September 18, 1996): 916–918.

Fairman, J. "Alternative Visions, The Nurse-Technology Relationship in the Context of the History of Technology." *Nursing History Review* 6 (1998): 129–146.

Fairman, Julie and Patricia D'Antonio "Virtual Power: Gendering the Nurse-Technology Relationship." *Nursing Inquiry* 6 (1999): 178–186.

Fye, W. Bruce. *American Cardiology: The History of a Specialty and its College*, Baltimore, MD: The John Hopkins University Press, 1996, 235.

Gerwig, Walter H. "The Surgical Intensive Care Unit." *Surgical Clinics of North America* 48 (August, 1968): 955–960.

Groeger et al., Jeffrey S. "Descriptive Analysis of Critical Care Units in the United States." *Critical Care Medicine* 20 (1992): 854.

Howell, Joel. *Technology in the Hospital: Transforming Patient Care in the Early Twentieth Century*. Baltimore, MD: John Hopkins, 1995.

Iberti, Thomas. J., Elaine K. Daily et al. "Assessment of Critical Care Nurses' Knowledge of the Pulmonary Artery Catheter." *Critical Care Medicine*, 22 (1994): 1674–1678.

Iberti, Thomas. J. et al. "A Multicenter Study of Physicians' Knowledge of the Pulmonary Artery Catheter." *Journal of American Medical Association* 264 (December 12, 1990): 2928–2932.

Lynaugh, Joan E. and Barbara L. Brush. *American Nursing: from Hospital to Health System*. Cambridge, MA: Blackwell Publishers, 1997.

Lynaugh, Joan E. and Julie A. Fairman. "New Nurses, New Spaces: A Preview of the AACN History Study." *American Journal of Critical Care* 1 (July 1992): 21.

Robin, Eugene D. "The Cult of the Swan-Ganz Catheter: Overuse and Abuse of Pulmonary Flow Catheters." *Annals of Internal Medicine* 103 (September 1985): 445–449.

Rogers, Everett M. *Diffusion of Innovations*, 4th ed. New York: The Free Press, 1995.

Romano, Carol A. "Predictors of Nurse Adoption of a Computerized Information System as an Innovation." *Medinformation* 2 (1995): 1335–1339.

Sandelowski, Margaret. "Making the Best of Things: Technology in American Nursing, 1870–1940." *Nursing History Review* 5 (1997): 3–22.

Sandelowski, Margaret. "The Physicians Eyes American Nursing and the Diagnostic Revolution in Medicine." *Nursing History Review* 8 (2000): 3–38.

Swan, H. J. C. "Balloon Flotation Catheters, Their Use in Hemodynamic Monitoring in Clinical Practice." *Journal of the American Medical Association* 233 (1975): 865–867.

Swan, H. J. C. and William Ganz. "Hemodynamic Monitoring: A Personal and Historical Perspective." *Canadian Medical Journal* 121 (October 6, 1979): 868–870.

_____."Hemodynamic Monitoring in Clinical Practice: A Decade in Review." *Journal of the American College of Cardiology* 1 (1983): 103–113.

Swan, H. J. C., William Ganz, James Forrester, Harold Marcus, George Diamond, and David Chonette. "Catheterization of the Heart in Man with Use of a Flow-Directed Balloon-Tipped Catheter." *New England Journal of Medicine* 283 (1970): 447–451.

Yehuda, Ginsor and Charles L. Sprung. "The Swan-Ganz Catheter, Twenty-Five Years of Monitoring." *Critical Care Clinics* 12 (1996): 771–776.

Zalumas, Jacqueline. *Caring In Crisis An Oral History of Critical Care Nursing*. Philadelphia, PA: University of Pennsylvania Press, 1995.

CHAPTER 11

Black Canadian Nurses and Technology

Karen Flynn

INTRODUCTION

Proficiency in the use of information and communication technology (ICT) by nurses in the new millennium is not only expected but also required. Nurses, for example, are expected to be computer literate, as care work is now done via the Internet or over the phone. Furthermore, ongoing implementation of E-health[1] initiatives will continue to fundamentally change how healthcare is delivered and subsequently how nurses define the scope of their practice. The ubiquitous presence of modern technology in healthcare has led to an uncritical acceptance of these systems and devices by clinicians. This, however, holds the potential to foreclose exploring technology's

[1]E-health may be defined as the combined use of information and communication technology (ICT) and electronic systems for various purposes, such as clinical (e.g., recording, retrieval, sharing, and maintaining patients' records), educational (e.g., training and learning by means of Internet and other electronic devices or through televideo consultation with the specialist doctors), research (e.g., evidence-based case studies, surveys, and trials), and administrative (e.g., identifying demographic indicators, trends of diseases, populations affected, policy decisions, implementation status query, etc.), which can be either at the local site or at distance in the health sector. See for example, Subhagata Chattopadhyay, "A Framework for Studying Perceptions of Rural Healthcare Staff and Basic ICT Support for e-Health Use: An Indian Experience," *Telemedicine and e-health* 16, no. 1 (January/February 2010): 80–88, doi:10.1089/tmj.2009.0081. See also, http://www.ehealthinitiative.org

complicated meanings. Reaction to the implementation of modern technology in nursing—as I will demonstrate—varies according to the historical context and the actors involved. An exploration of how practitioners initially grappled with the introduction of technology into nursing provides a context to understand current debates around its practice and use.

As part of a larger research project on black Canadian and Caribbean immigrant women in Canada, this chapter is based on interviews of 35 nurses from 1995 to 2007 regarding their childhood, nursing education and training, family, work, and community, among other themes.[2] The objective is to map black nurses' conflicting and contested relationship to technology while being attentive to their social location—that is, how they were situated within nursing. The exclusionary practices of nursing schools and the Department of Citizenship and Immigration meant that in the world of post–World War II nursing in Canada, black practitioners were the exception rather than the rule. Black nurses worked alongside a primarily white clinical staff within a culture that reinforced whiteness and white cultural practices and norms. Notwithstanding the fact that the interviewees identified themselves as nurses—and not as *black* nurses—they remained far from oblivious to the fact their blackness was not always invisible to other clinical personnel and patients. Subsequently, black nurses' response to technology is not only intricately connected to economic, social, and political processes but is also a tacit mindfulness of how their own raced bodies might be read.

Gender then cannot be the sole or primary analytical paradigm used to articulate social relationships in healthcare. In doing so, we run the risk of underestimating the myriad and complex ways in which structures of power produce and reproduce social divisions in the workplace, not only among physicians and nurses, but also between nurses. Though black nurses remain differentiated by education, age, training, time of migration, and other factors, incorporating their voices as knowing and self-reflective subjects in the discussion of technology not only allows for a polyvocality of perspectives but also serves to legitimize their knowledge. Simply put, including black practitioners' perspectives renders a more dynamic reading and interpretation of nursing relationship to technology.

---

[2]See Karen Flynn, *Beyond Borders: Moving beyond Borders: Black Canadian and Caribbean Women in the African Diaspora* (University of Toronto Press, forthcoming). In addition to signing consent forms, the interviewees were also given the option of using pseudonyms; only four of the women chose this option. The tapes are currently in the possession of the author.

Generally speaking, when feminist scholars conceptualize the meaning of technology for women in relation to paid work in North America, they either view technology as reinforcing social inequality—that is, women are viewed as victims of technology—or they see technology as a mixed blessing. For the first group, a major concern is how technology reinforces and maintains social inequality, based on race, class, gender, age, or other markers of difference. Eileen B. Leonard, for example, points out that "for many women workers, developing technologies have yet to deliver as promised . . . . it has done little to improve the status of women in the workplace."[3] Furthermore, she continues, women of color are often concentrated in "labor-intensive, low technology work."[4] Alternatively, those who view technology as a "mixed blessing" caution against a reductionist and positivist view of women's relationship to technology. Instead of accepting that technology automatically means progress, it is important to explore how it contributes to the creation of a sexual division of labor, but also how this division of labor is dismantled and re-established through individual and collective efforts.[5]

Larger feminist debates about women and technology also resonate within nursing. Nursing scholars undoubtedly concur that the introduction of technology into nursing has substantially restructured the physical aspect of the occupation and has affected how patient care is administered.[6] For example, American nursing scholar Margarete Sandelowski, in *Devices and Desires: Gender, Technology, and American Nursing*, noted that introduction of new technologies operated simultaneously to impede and benefit nurses. Nursing scholar Ruth Minard remains less optimistic. Even though nurses gain new skills to operate new technologies, she argues, there is the fear that such technologies actually deskills them because they detract from the caring aspect of nursing which is fundamental to the occupation. In the long run, Minard intimates, technology drains the skill requirements, resulting in a demand for semi skilled rather than skilled workers. Furthermore, she continues, "Technology is not confined to the introduction of machines, but includes changes at

---

[3]Eileen B. Leonard, *Women, Technology, and the Myth of Progress* (New Jersey: Prentice Hall, 2003), 116; See also selected chapters in Mary Frank Fox, Deborah G. Johnson, and Sue V. Rosser, eds., *Women, Gender, and Technology* (Urbana, IL: University of Illinois, Press).

[4]Leonard, *Women, Technology, and the Myth of Progress*, 118.

[5]See, for example, Juliet Webster, *Shaping Women's Work: Gender, Employment and Information Technology* (New York: Longman Sociology Press, 1996).

[6]For a contemporary discussion see, Margarete Sandelowski, "Visible Humans, Vanishing Bodies, and Virtual Nursing: Complications of Life, Presence, Place, and Identity," *Advance Nursing Science* 24, no. 3 (2002): 58–70.

the site of production, in the transfer of production between the workstations, and in the coordination of the two."[7] Rinard further equates the increase in the numbers and types and use of drugs by nurses to the introduction of machines in manufacturing. In contrast, Julie A. Fairman offers an alternative view of nurses' relationship to technology that moves beyond the traditional machine/human dyad. She pushes instead for an analysis that is grounded in history and context, further proposing that we understand technology as socially constructed rather than as some abstract entity that remains disconnected from political, social, and economic processes.[8] Drawing on Fairman's analyses, this chapter explores black nurses' responses to technology from the perspective of nurses who were retired, nearing retirement, and those who were still employed at the time of the interview.

TECHNOLOGICAL TERRAIN

Once black Canadian nurses gained formal admittance to train and work in Canada's nursing schools and hospitals beginning in the early 1950s, they entered a field undergoing rapid technological, diagnostic, and surgical transformations. In addition, the introduction of myriad new drugs was also common. In some ways, the occupation benefited from these changes as nurses ventured into male-dominated terrain. Once the purview of physicians, tasks such as taking blood pressure and starting intravenous drips were relinquished to RNs. Technological changes accelerated into the twenty-first century. Increased electronic machinery and specialized care units such as the intensive care unit (ICU) characterized the mid-1950s to the 1980s. Moreover, as a way to control both cost and care, new technologies were implemented in the 1980s and 1990s. Undoubtedly, similar patterns existed in Britain where most of the Caribbean nurses trained. Of course, by the mid-1970s, the Caribbean migrant nurses discussed in this study had already migrated to Canada. Indeed, these nurses who entered the occupation during the early 1950s to the 1970s had to reconcile traditional nursing values with the introduction of modern technology.

---

[7]Ruth G. Minard, "Technology, Deskilling and Nurses: The Impact of the Technologically Changing Environment," *Advances in Nursing Science* 18, no. 4 (1996): 62.
[8]Julie A. Fairman, "Alternative Visions: The Nurse-Technology Relationship in the Context of the History of Technology," *Nursing History Review* 6 (1998): 129–146.

How black nurses articulated their reaction to technology cannot be attributed to any single factor. Indeed, for black Canadian-born and Caribbean-migrant nurses, their presence as racialized women is but one factor. Nurses who trained in the British system, whether in the Caribbean or Britain, and who migrated to Canada mostly during the 1960s to the 1970s, felt that their training, knowledge, and skills superseded that of their Canadian counterparts. Consequently, their discussion of technology is integrally connected to how they positioned themselves vis-a-vis Canadian nurses regardless of color. black Canadian nurses, on the other hand, understood the intrusion of technology as not only inevitable, given transformations in the healthcare field, but also in some cases vital.

Black nurses in this study were cognizant of the fact that the introduction of technology had implications for how they performed their duties. Still, none of the nurses expressed an outright aversion to technology. Of the two groups, black Canadians expressed more optimism about its use. They advocated and applauded the use of technology as long as patient care was not compromised and if there were actual improvements at the bedside. Caribbean migrant nurses, on the other hand, while conscious of how technology extended the range of nurses' work (from which some of them benefited), were less laudatory than their Canadian counterparts. Consequently, there was some conjecture about how technology not only altered nurses' work, but also relationships between nurses.

As racialized women working in predominantly white spaces, some nurses acquired training in specialized areas where demands for technological skills were valued, and consequently they gained more respect. Besides developing new skills, the interviewees also mentioned other advantages, including accepting the challenges of a new unit, autonomy, a more egalitarian relationship with physicians, and the opportunity to develop their confidence in a given area. Throughout their careers, some of the nurses were employed in the emergency room (ER), operating room (OR), hemodialysis unit, the ICU, and cardiology.

An RN with midwifery training, Inez Mackenzie, immigrated to Ontario from Jamaica during the 1960s where she worked in pediatrics for almost a decade. Mackenize wanted a new challenge in a more specialized area, so she enrolled at Humber College in Ontario. For Mackenize, the OR was a more ideal site because it demanded greater technical skills and knowledge. At the same time, as a proponent of specialization, Mackenzie was not only interested in the challenge these units present for nurses, but also underscored how patients benefit:

> It is good to specialize. I am thinking of intensive care. There was a time when you could go in intensive care and rotate whereas you probably didn't

> like intensive care; you just go because you are sent there because there is an opening. I find the more you specialize is the more care you give because that is your personal choice, so you are able to do more for the patient then.[9]

For nurses such as Mackenzie, technology is viewed in a dialectical manner. Thus, when nurses make decisions regarding the extent of their involvement in specialized areas that demand increased technological aptitude, they are hardly passive recipients of technology. Moreover, Mackenzie's inclusion of patients in her rationale speaks to their centrality as important subjects critical to any discussion about technology.

Notwithstanding the fact that black nurses all trained in the apprenticeship system, those trained in the Caribbean and Britain felt the training far exceeded that of their Canadian counterparts. Upon migrating to Canada, the majority of interviewees found that tasks that they had been responsible for in the Caribbean and Britain remained in the physicians' domain. This was especially so for nurse-midwives. Barbadian-born, British-trained Muriel Knight noted that upon arrival in Canada also in 1960:

> There were a lot [of] skills (such as giving aspirins to patients) being done by physicians that was [sic] being done by nurses in England and the Caribbean. Inserting a tube in somebody's nose and their stomach was what I did as a second year nursing student. And I couldn't do that as a nurse when I came here.[10]

Indeed, wanting to capture some aspect of the professional life left behind might also explain why some Caribbean nurses chose more specialized and technologically driven areas where they were able to utilize the knowledge and skills from their previous training. For example, nurses who worked in high-intensity areas such as the ICU and the ER felt that physicians valued their input and expertise, which added to their confidence. They also emphasized the mutual respect that existed between nurses and physicians.

When she migrated to Ontario in the early 1970s, Jamaican-born British-trained Dorette Thompson first worked in the hemodialysis unit and several years later took the necessary courses that enabled her to move to the ER. For Thompson, nursing encompassed more than managing the technology that necessitates the smooth functioning of the unit:

---

[9]Inez Mackenzie, tape-recorded interview by author, Markham, Ontario, October 13, 1999.

[10]Muriel Knight, tape-recorded interview by author, Scarborough, Ontario, September 9, 2006.

> Nurses are more autonomous and you have responsibilities, and the fact that you work alongside the doctor [who] relies on you like in Emerg and Hemo . . . that's why I like those areas . . . the doctor relies on us a lot because we know the patient, they don't. And that's the good thing about the areas that I'm working in now [;] it's where I get the satisfaction.[11]

Other nurses such as Knight who already had experience working in the ER department in Britain and the casualty unit (similar to the ER) in Barbados also expressed a profound sense of satisfaction working in the ER in Canada. In addition to discussing how important it was for her to be as, or even more, knowledgeable than the physician, Knight also highlighted the reciprocal relationship that existed between physicians and nurses.

Fairman's contention that any discussion about technology is narrow when the primary focus is fixed on machines, and their function is certainly applicable to Caribbean migrant nurses. When these interviewees made decisions about upgrading into critical care nursing, they did not act on impulse but weighed their options carefully. That is, they took into consideration multiple factors. Certainly, the prestige was one reason, but there were also the social relationships—especially with physicians—coupled with their own skills and ability. Like some of their Caribbean counterparts, a few of the black Canadian interviewees also worked in coronary care units where they navigated their roles with machines used to diagnose patients.

TECHNOLOGY AND ITS BENEFITS FOR BLACK CANADIAN NURSES

Canadian-born Marlene Watson first worked as an RN in the recovery unit at Toronto Western Hospital in Ontario during the early 1960s. Watson graduated from Victoria General Hospital in Halifax, Nova Scotia, in 1961 and moved to Toronto immediately thereafter. She left Toronto Western in the mid-1970s to work in the ICU at the York Finch Hospital in North York, Ontario. To improve efficiency and cut costs, York Finch configured the ICU to include coronary care, postcoronary care, endocrinology, and gastroenterology; and Watson rose to a supervisory position in the mid-1980s. Drawing on her extensive nursing and supervisory positions in these specialized areas, Watson explained that in many respects, "technology has been great, and I think it

---

[11]Dorrette Thompson [pseudonym] tape-recorded interview by author, Scarborough, Ontario, August 17, 1999.

offers a whole lot more of nurses' 'interpretation of patients' wellness . . ."[12] To support her point, Watson used the example of a patient who underwent open-heart surgery. In a situation such as this, Watson maintained, a highly experienced and skilled nurse would look after the patient. This nurse, she continued, would be able to examine the monitor the patient is hooked up to and "see if they are going to fibulate . . . You could be forewarned because you have a nurse sitting there responsible [for] checking those monitors as they go along." Of course, one can argue that Watson's mention of the "nurse sitting there" is precisely the issue with some aspects of technology. Some of it could be monotonous, repetitive, and boring.

From Watson's and other nurses' vantage point, *they* used technology, it did not use *them*. That is, they were not dupes who naively assumed that modern technology and scientific advances would resolve all medical troubles, but they recognized the advantages. Some nurses, including Watson, felt that patients profited the most from technology. To elucidate her argument, Watson hearkened back to an earlier period in her training before the introduction of certain technological devices, such as the tympanic thermometer[13] which was introduced during the mid-1980s:

> We don't have patients biting thermometers and cracking them in their mouths, [since] we had oral thermometers. Now we get a needle [probe], and we can just stick them in the ear, and in two seconds the temperature is taken. It [technology] has taken the danger aspect away as well.

In tandem with prompt and accurate diagnosis, technology helped to protect patients from unnecessary harms.

Viewed as an efficiency-saving mechanism, certain technological devices ultimately meant the saving of lives. Frieda Steele, another black Canadian-born nurse who graduated from Hotel Dieu in Windsor, Ontario, in 1950, noted that "we can get reports right away; we don't have to rely on invasive surgery for answers. It [technology] is fast and efficient."[14] References were made to how specimen tests produced more accurate results and were done at a much faster pace than the older method. One such older method involved nurses testing urine samples on the hospital unit, using special plastic and paper test strips, where estimates were made about the amount of chemicals in the urine, such as glucose, blood, or proteins. These tests relied on nurses' visual comparison of color results. With the new technology, the tests were

---

[12]Marlene Watson, tape-recorded interview by author, Toronto, Ontario, January 18, 2000.
[13]Thanks to Cynthia Toman for her technological expertise.
[14]Frieda Parker Steele, tape-recorded interview by author, Windsor, Ontario, June 9, 2001.

done in the labs by machines, which guaranteed a much higher degree of accuracy rates.[15] Watson and other black Canadian nurses pointed out that nurses in critical care units who were well trained to operate the machines could assess their patients more intelligently. The use of certain technology further prevented the overcrowding of certain departments, another benefit to patients and nurses alike. Drawing again on the example of the patient who had a surgical operation, Watson pointed out, "we whip them into the recovery room, and most recovery rooms can take a respirator," which then freed up space for other postoperative patients.

Watson's and Steele's optimism about technology and patient care was sometimes interrupted by further introspection as they contemplated their overall perception of the various devices upon which nurses relied. Steele mentioned, for example, how technology affected nurses' skills—skills that remain intrinsic to how nurses care for their patients. She explained:

> I think that the observation skills of nurses have been downgraded. I feel that the nurses don't have time, and doctors don't seem to listen or rely on them like they used to. The machines are not able to tell us, for example, that Mrs. Jones is worried about a sick child at home, or that she is worried about leaving her ailing mother at home.

Referred to as the "psychological aspect of caring" by a Caribbean nurse, Steele recognized that nurses, not diagnostic machines, were best able to satisfy the emotional needs of some patients. Regardless of the ubiquitous presence of technology in the field of healthcare, it can never replace some of the vital functions performed by nurses.

Watson insisted that once nurses were trained to operate a particular technology, it was easier to make more intelligent decisions with respect to patient care. But she also acknowledged that sitting in a room for 8 hours observing a machine did not encompass all that a nurse was trained to do. Furthermore, in a situation where a nurse was monitoring a patient from a different location it was difficult to simultaneously use technology and provide "hands-on" patient care. Thus, there was some recognition that practitioners who monitor devices were being deskilled because this work can be monotonous, unchallenging, and render obsolete other abilities that are central to nursing. How both groups of black Canadian nurses conceptualize technology was far from reductionist. They aptly weighed the advantages and disadvantages of the various technological devices and their relationship to them.

---

[15]See, for example, Joel D. Howell, *Technology in the Hospital: Transforming Patient Care in the Early Twentieth Century* (The Johns Hopkins University Press, 1995).

TECHNOLOGY AND ITS LIMITATIONS FOR BLACK BRITISH AND CARIBBEAN NURSES

Unlike the black Canadian interviewees, Caribbean nurses' discussion of technology was more encompassing. These nurses situated their discussion of technology within the broader political economy of healthcare in tandem with how they as migrants viewed the Canadian healthcare system. Indeed, they, too, acknowledged the advantages of technological and scientific advances within healthcare. Yet Caribbean nurses were not always convinced that the quality of patient care improved, especially at the end of their careers with the restructuring of the Canadian healthcare system. While they could not alter the inevitability of technological interventions in nursing, these practitioners hardly accepted these devices passively. Rita Maloney, paraphrasing educator and scholar Marie Campbell, points out that "technology continually transforms the context and ideas people use to think about it, making it difficult for nurses or anyone else to stand back and judge its impact. But nurses must stand back and judge."[16] Indeed, Caribbean nurses' articulation of technology suggests that they *did* more than standing back and judging.

Trained in Jamaica, June Heaven migrated to Northern British Columbia in 1967. Seven months later she left for Ontario, where she worked for a short time at two different hospitals. She then left Toronto for Ottawa to complete her baccalaureate degree in nursing in 1969, while working as a team leader at the Centenary Hospital. Heaven returned to Toronto and began teaching at Humber College in 1971 (she also completed a master's degree during this time) through her retirement in the mid-1990s. Heaven's discussion of technology thus adopts the perspective of both a nurse and a nurse educator.

For this interviewee, debates about technology and the effect on patient care requires contextualization. That is, how technology is deployed is intricately connected to how the wider society sees and values the role of caring. For Heaven, changes in nursing education and the concomitant skills that nurses have acquired have benefited the discipline as a whole. "Without a doubt, nurses have required more skills with high-tech procedures. You have better-educated nurses to handle more high-tech procedures," she remarked. Yet, Heaven expressed some concerns. She saw a connection between technological advancement, working conditions, and society's overall attitude about caring, links that ultimately affect the patient. Heaven noted that during the early 1990s the patient/nurse ratio was much higher than in previous

---

[16]Rita Maloney, "Technological Issues," in *Canadian Nursing Face The Future,* eds. Alice J. Baumgart and Jenniece Larsen, 2nd ed. (Toronto, ON: Mosby Year Book, 1991), 295.

years, which affected not only nurses' well-being but also how patient care was delivered. She further posited that we currently live in a society that is indifferent, and she argued that technological advancement contributes to this process as nurses come to depend on machines and caring takes a secondary role. According to Heaven, "People are coming into nursing from a society where caring is less." For Heaven, then, increased technology usage cannot be understood in isolation from the changes taking place in society, and, by extension nursing. Thus, her conceptualization echoes Susan Reverby's often-repeated stance that "nursing is a form of labour shaped by the order to care in a society that refuses to value caring."[17]

Caribbean interviewees also spoke critically of how the implementation of technology in nursing created divisions between differently situated nurses. In this scenario, Heaven (who is a nursing educator) and specialized nurses (those with technological skills) might view the bedside as the prerogative of less well-trained nurses. Surely, some nurses acquired technological expertise to distinguish themselves from other practitioners while removing themselves from the bedside, however the Caribbean- and British-trained nurses interviewed did not express this motivation. They continually emphasized the significance of patient care, which they found lacking upon migration to Canada.

British- and Caribbean-trained nurses were hardly reticent in their criticisms of their Canadian counterparts regardless of color. One area in which they found their Canadian counterparts lacking was in ministering to the needs of their patients. Though both groups trained in hospital-based nursing schools, Caribbean nurses felt that their practical and theoretical training put them at an advantage. They also pointed out that training was more comprehensive, which allowed them to care for multiple patients at any given time, compared to their Canadian nurses, who could only manage, for example, three patients. Finally, a few Caribbean nurses suggested that that they placed more value on patient care, which they saw as critical given the transformations occurring in nursing.

Jamaican-born, British-trained nurse-midwife Daphne Bailey immigrated to Brantford, Ontario, in 1960. She worked at Brantford Hospital for 2 years before leaving for Toronto where she worked at Doctors Hospital for 8 years. She then completed a certificate in public health at the University of Toronto and subsequently found employment in 1971 with the Victoria Order of Nurses (VON), an organization that provides in-home nursing care. During the 25 1/2 years that Bailey worked with the VON, she earned a BA and several

---

[17]Susan Reverby, *Ordered to Care: The Dilemma of American Nursing 1850–1945* (New York: Cambridge of University, 1987), 1.

certificates, taking courses, that she felt "would help me with the VON." Among her multiple positions Bailey also worked as an intravenous (IV) nurse, another specialty area.

Bailey insisted that black nurses valued caring more so than white nurses did. She noted that black nurses were kinder, more empathetic, and had a more holistic way of viewing the patient. "We were taught to look after the whole patient," Bailey points out. Bailey attributed this difference in caring to Caribbean nurses' religious upbringing and sense of community, a perspective that she felt that was corroborated by white patients when she worked in England and Canada. "I think we have a more caring spirit [sic]. When I came here [referring to Canada], I found it very difficult, the nurses had their own little patient, and if your patient wanted water, they would say "I'm not your nurse."[18] While working as an IV nurse, Bailey noticed that "the nurses would leave the tray [while] the patients are lying flat. They didn't raise the bed or anything." She would then go around "raise the bed and put the trays in front of them [patients]," tasks that were normally the auxiliary staff's responsibility. Compared to many other black and white nurses, Bailey was not only more educated, but also had more experience, yet this did not preclude her from being attentive to the basic needs of the patients.

British-trained, Grenadian-born Dorothy Jones also migrated to Canada during the 1960s and worked as a registered nursing assistant (RNA). She later went back to school to become an RN. For Jones, technology appeared to be replacing traditional nurses' knowledge, especially among newer nursing graduates. Missing from nursing in the 1990s, she felt, was a system whereby older, more experienced nurses acted as mentors for younger nurses passing on their knowledge as opposed to giving machines precedence over nurses' experience. An aspect of this knowledge to which Jones referred was the practical aspect of nurse training that she perceives Canadian nurses, especially those trained in colleges, might not have received. Here she explained:

> The younger people are just graduating and coming in, they don't have the older nurses to prime them, you know, to pass on their experience. But with the new technology, they do everything by the computer, but the basic hard working experience that the older nurses had, you wouldn't find that among the new nurses coming in. So in that way it's more or less left for computers and machines . . . .[19]

---

[18]Daphne Bailey, tape-recorded interview by author, Toronto, Ontario, May 5, 1995.
[19]Dorothy Jones, [pseudonym], tape-recorded interview by author, Rexdale, Ontario, February 29, 2000.

According to her, the older nurses were "just holding on, doing the best that they could, they are waiting to get out."

RESTRUCTURING AND TECHNOLOGY

Interestingly enough, while the interviewees generally accepted the use of technology such as cardiac machines and respirators in critical care units, they were especially critical of computers. The introduction of computerized systems was seen as more of a nuisance due to their time-consuming nature. Generational differences between the two groups of nurses further accounted for how each viewed and employed computer technology. Essentially, those nurses who began working in the 1950s and 1960s displayed more discomfort with the use of computers in the hospitals than those who were still working at the time of the interview. The former mostly saw it as greatly impeding bedside care, while the latter viewed computers as part of the transformation the healthcare field was undergoing. It appeared, one interviewee from the first group lamented, "that nurses spend more time putting things in the computer, and trying to work this computer." That most of these nurses were much older and not accustomed to using computers undoubtedly made the task much more difficult. Mackenzie further explained that due to "a lot of documentation . . . you find that sometimes you have not done enough for the patient physically." She added, however, that despite the excess use of computers, that patients and nurses were protected in the event of a legal dispute. Clearly, nurses such as Mackenzie are watching and judging; they did not use these technologies uncritically.

While the interviewees pointed to the time-consuming nature of computers, Canadian nursing researcher Jacqueline Choniere maintains that computerized systems are often accompanied by new management protocols in an effort to manage the workplace. Speaking specifically about the computerized patient classification system implemented in the 1970s and 1980s, Choniere argues that:

> Management, in an effort to rationalize the workplace, had created a new work organization to enhance the new technology. More specifically, management had found a technology which they believed would help them to rationalize the workplace. The new technology supports the new organization, and the resulting changes in the nature of work exert pressure on the worker, in an attempt to prevent her from functioning as before.[20]

---

[20]Jacqueline Choiniere, "A Case Study Examination of Nurses and Patient Information Technology," in *Vital Signs: Nursing Work in Transition,* eds. Pat Armstrong, Jacqueline Choiniere and Elaine Day (Toronto, ON: Garamound Press, 1993), 66.

The end result, Campbell argues, was that "a scarcity of time orientation was programmed into nurses' thinking about caring, through their involvement in classifying patients in units of time needed for care."[21] Essentially, nurses were forced to rethink how they managed patient care.

If the implementation of computerized technology in hospitals was one way for management to control nurses' labor, this did not always have the desired effect. Nurses were not always compliant subjects. Watson, for example, avoided using the computer, finding other ways such as the telephone to communicate when she needed to. Watson insisted:

> I don't even bother with the computer . . . By the time I type in I.D.'s and all that stuff; I could have done another I.V. By the time I get done with this information input and then I have to do my charting afterward, I find that for me it does not save me any time. If I had my own way, I would probably do away with computers.

Clearly, Watson and some of her counterparts astutely assessed the ineffectiveness of various forms of technology instituted in the workplace. Moreover, nurses who, like Watson, figured out how to avoid using the computer exercised some form of agency.

Technology and Cost Containment

As illustrated thus far, black Canadian and Caribbean nurses recognized that not only did technology offer nurses' options, it also reinforced their claims to professionalism as skilled and knowledgeable workers. At the same time, the structural and organizational changes hospitals made during the 1990s as a part of larger healthcare reforms in Canada led the interviewees who were still working during this time to conclude that hospitals had their own agenda, which did not always include them or the patients. Thus, technological systems were thus bound up in efforts to reduce expenditures. While some nurses tried their utmost to resist the encroachment of certain forms of technology upon their daily work, this was a difficult endeavor.

Trained in Canada during the 1970s, Jamaican-born Janet Barrett explained how some technology instituted by hospitals not only increased profits, but also allowed management to reduce the number of nursing personnel. Barrett used the following example to illustrate her point:

---

[21]Marie Campbell, "Knowledge, Gendered Subjectivity, and the Restructuring of HealthCare: The Case of the Disappearing Nurse," in *Restructuring Caring Labour: Discourse, State Practice, and Everyday Life*, ed. Sheila M. Neysmith (Toronto, ON: Oxford University Press, 2000), 190.

> [Before] when you [took] a temperature you had to stand there and wait for the thermometer to reach its level. Now in seconds, you can do the temperature. Because the technology wasn't there you had more time then to spend with the patient. They have cut the staff in nursing because they [management] are saying it's taking less time to do the things you used to do. The patient interaction is no longer there like it used to be.[22]

For Barrett, management deliberately engaged in the centralization of work to control the labor process at the expense of healthcare workers and patients. Hence, "to restructure the delivery of patient services and inject it with more of the vigor of the market means organizing caregivers to do their work differently."[23]

In the midst of cutbacks, short staffing, and stagnant wages, black nurses found themselves questioning the very philosophy and foundation on which nursing has been constructed. For those interviewees who were still employed, the ability and desire to "care" had certainly been eroded. Hospitals, they felt, had adopted a business-like model, that remained antiethical to patient care. Here, another interviewee illuminated the following:

> Hospitals run like businesses and nurses are at the bottom of the totem pole. They know that nurses will work anyway, because you can't walk off a unit and abandon your patients. They cash in the whole philosophy of what a nurse does, the caring, nurturing, so you are going to continue nursing. We are held hostage to that.

This interviewee clearly recognized nurses' vulnerability as hospitals implemented strategies to compete in what had become an "increasingly market- or quasi-market-oriented healthcare system."[24]

Once the beneficiaries of modern technology—at least in the beginning of its implementation—hospital restructuring ultimately affected how patient care was administered. Brenda Lewis earned her RN diploma in psychiatric nursing in Trinidad, but upon migration to Canada in the early 1970s found out that her diploma was not recognized by the College of Nursing. Subsequently, she, too, earned her registered nursing licensure. Lewis had this to say:

> You don't have time to do that [patient care] now. You have got to do your paper work and you have so many patients to look after, before you had less, and you could really do bedside nursing for your patients. But now it's a matter of survival, of getting the workload done. So you cut corners to survive.[25]

---

[22]Janet Barrett, [pseudonym] tape-recorded interview by author, Toronto, Ontario, June 5, 2000.

[23]Campbell, "Knowledge, Gendered Subjectivity, and the Restructuring of HealthCare," 188.

[24]Ibid.

[25]Brenda Lewis, tape-recorded interview by author, Toronto, Ontario, February 24, 2000.

The use of new technology not only reorganized the daily routine of nurses' work, but also affected social relationships between nurses and their superiors. While Caribbean nurses tended to overlook the skill and educational differences between themselves and the ancillary staff, this did not always extend to supervisors. Indeed, nurse managers were often in a conflicted position as those responsible for ensuring that the new technologies and management systems were being implemented. Canadian nursing scholars Alice Baumgart and Jenniece Larsen argued that "nurses who occupy middle-management positions are often laden with budget, staffing and related functions as a result of decentralization and frequently have very little time to provide necessary 'support work' to ensure that nurses feel valued [or] will take risks to find out creative solutions to workplace problems."[26] Thompson offered her insight into how management has changed in the past 20 years in a way that reaffirmed Baumgart and Larsen's analysis. According to Thompson, management showed very little interest in the welfare of workers, and her frustration was evident:

> Managers used to care about you. You are not well, just go home. People would care and you would get your vacation. Now I can't even get a vacation this year because we don't have enough staff, and they can't grant you vacation, if they don't have any staff. Nurses are caught in a catch twenty-two because we work in the healthcare field and caring for people whose lives are in your hand, you can't take a vacation because there is no staff.

CONCLUSION

Indeed, clinicians working in healthcare in the millennium have accepted the ongoing technologization of healthcare as normal. For black Canadian nurses who entered nurse training during the late 1940s and 1950s and their Caribbean counterparts who joined them during the 1960s and 1970s, modern technology drastically transformed and expanded their scope of practice. Black Canadian nurses generally felt that patients gained the most as a result of modern technology. Caribbean nurses, on the other hand, remained more tentative, especially in their analysis. This was mostly evident in the case of nurses who were still working at the time of the interview and had to deal

---

[26]Alice J. Baumgart and Jenniece Larsen, eds., *Canadian Nurses Faces the Future*, 2nd ed. (Toronto, ON: Mosby Year Book, 1992), 233–234.

with the effects of restructuring. Even though there were some nurses who actually acquired certain skills and training that placed them in areas that demanded technological expertise, this did not mean they acquiesced to the changes wrought by technology. Caribbean nurses interviewed insist that technology cannot be divorced from the political economy of healthcare. Cost-containment measures proposed and implemented beginning in the 1970s and 1980s, and the restructuring of healthcare in the 1990s, has led to disillusionment among nurses who were still working at the time of the interviews. Whether they were trained in the Caribbean, Britain, or Canada, black nurses did not view themselves as victims of technology, or that technology automatically meant progress. What the interviews reveal is that discussions about technology have to be contextualized and placed within a political, economical, and social context. In doing so, black healthcare professionals emerge not as victims of technology, but as active agents who were able to navigate a contested terrain while ensuring that patient care was rarely compromised.

ACKNOWLEDGMENTS

I thank Cynthia Toman for her technological expertise, and I also thank Meryn Stuart and Jayne Elliott.

Section IV

NURSING INTERVENTIONS: NEGOTIATING SPACE

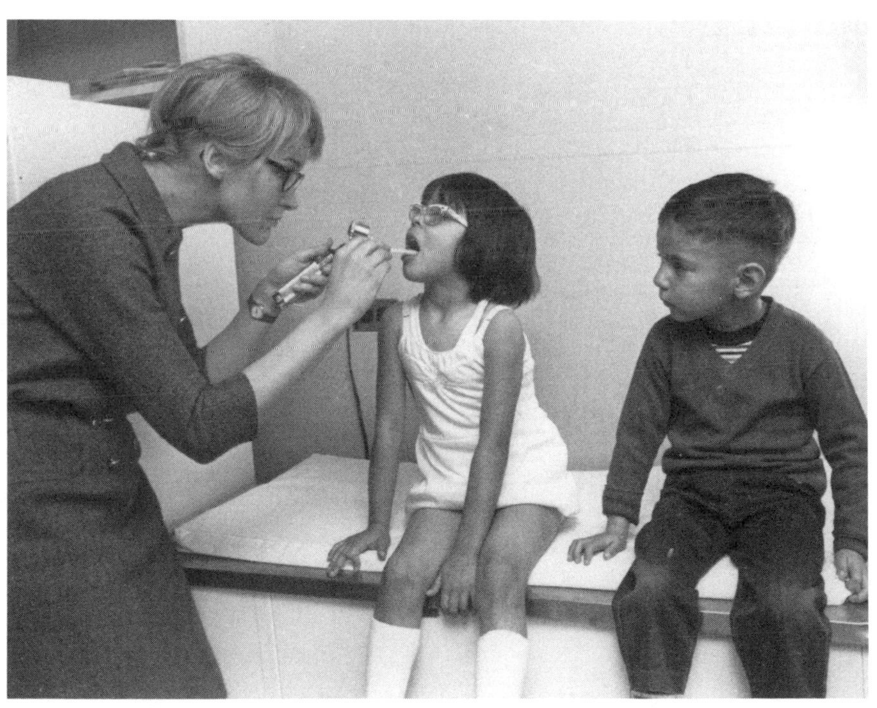

CHAPTER 12

To Avoid Expense and Suffering: Public Health Nurses and the Struggle for Health Services

Rima D. Apple

INTRODUCTION

Today's Nurse–Family Partnership Program (NFP) is

> . . . an evidence-based program that aims to improve the lives of at-risk, first-time mothers and their infants. The program pairs these women with specially trained nurses, who conduct home visits for roughly two and a half years, beginning before the birth of the infant.[1]

This description reads very much like that of the Director of the Wisconsin Bureau of Maternal and Child Health (MCH) who, nearly 70 years earlier, explained that

> . . . a public health nurse . . . can make family contacts with expectant mothers and infants, thus carrying a health education program directly into the homes. . . . this program will make a very real contribution to the conservation of lives of mothers and children and also aid in establishing health early for the children. . . .[2]

---

[1]Katy Dawley, Joan Loch, and Irene Bindrich, "The Nurse-Family Partnership," *American Journal of Nursing* 107, no. 11 (2007): 60–63.

[2]Amy Louise Hunter, "Letter to Ed Jensen, Chairman, Barron County Board of Supervisors. 9 February 1940," in *Wisconsin Bureau of Maternal and Child Health, Programs and demonstrations, 1922–1961* (Madison, WI: Wisconsin State Historical Society) [hereafter referred to as *M&CH*] box 11, folder 10.

As the NFP nurses do, MCH nurses recognized the need for health education in the homes of new mothers and infants. But, their goal was more ambitious: They expected to convince local governments that a public health nurse was a vital component of county affairs. An MCH nurse was successful when the county board took on the financial commitment for the program. The history of the MCH program documents health, economic, political, and cultural factors that influenced the shape of public health practices yesterday and the pivotal role that nurses played and continue to play today in the development of public health efforts.

EARLY COUNTY PUBLIC HEALTH EFFORTS IN WISCONSIN

In the early twentieth century, high infant and maternal mortality rates raised concern in many parts of the country. In addition, World War I examinations of soldiers disclosed numerous cases of ill health that analysts believed could have been prevented with appropriate medical oversight in childhood. States blamed the lack of attention to the health of infants and children on maternal ignorance and they developed different means to ameliorate the problem.[3] In the 1920s, Wisconsin sent nurses in "Well-Child Trailers" into rural areas to conduct talks on maternal and child health. The bureau quickly realized this "classroom" education was not enough. Subsequently, the MCH established a series of roaming health centers at which children were weighed, measured, and examined by a bureau physician who then told the mother the health status of her child, directed her to a local physician if the child needed treatment, and reminded the mother of the importance of regular checkups by her private physician.[4]

Centers were hugely successful. Many rural mothers who lacked access to private physicians brought their children to the centers to learn about diet, sanitation, and the like, and to have a physician examine their children.

---

[3]For more on mothers in this period, see Rima D. Apple, *Perfect Motherhood: Science and Childrearing in America* (New Brunswick, NJ: Rutgers University Press, 2006).

[4]Information about the goals and practices of the Child Health Centers may be found in *M&CH,* box 3, folder 3. Information about the audiences for these centers is found scattered through the various reports sent to the state bureaus. Many of these are now located in *M&CH,* box 16, folder 2 and box 6, folder 5. Remember that in the United States there is an attempt to clearly distinguish between public health and private medicine. Bureau staff were keenly aware of the problems they would have with local physicians if they were seen to be usurping the role of the private doctors. Therefore, the centers educated, they examined, they directed mothers to physicians; but they did not treat.

Center staff was pleased with the results. Dr. Eleanor Hutchinson proudly reported that the August 20, 1930, center in Barron, Wisconsin

> had 42 at the clinic. We had several of the older ones who have not attended for 2 years or more. There were several improvements in the way of tonsils, teeth, and so on, also vaccinations . . . . People drive for a good number of miles to attend these clinics and the interest has been excellent.[5]

Repeat visits proved to the State Board of Health that families learned the importance of regular medical supervision.[6]

However, repeat attendees pointed to three critical problems. First, conducting centers once or twice a year provided only limited continuity of care. By the 1940s, follow-up was so vital that the bureau would refuse to establish centers in counties without public health nurses who could ensure that mothers followed the directions they were given, especially when that advice involved referrals to local physicians. Second was the difficulty in accessing local doctors. Physicians were happy when centers referred patients to them for treatment, but in this time period, rural Wisconsin doctors rarely thought in terms of preventive medicine. Moreover, in many cases patients could not afford physicians, and local physicians were not inclined to make nonemergency house calls when families lived outside of town on barely maintained dirt roads. Third, and most significant, centers were just that, centers. They were held in a central location and families traveled to them. Center staff had little or no idea about the home conditions and other family factors that affected children's health. Only home visits could determine the economic circumstances, the housing conditions, and other environmental factors that affected the family's health. Centers were neither prepared nor able to collect such vital information.

These limitations frustrated MCH staff. They acknowledged that there seemed to be a great need for centers; but, in counties without county nurses it was impossible to follow up the defects found, to ensure that mothers understood the directions of the state physicians, to identify other sources of ill health, and to prod mothers to attend local physicians for needed treatments.[7]

---

[5]Eleanor Hutchinson, "Report from Barron, 20 August 1930," in *M&CH,* box 6, folder 5, 6.
[6]The bureau staff rarely questioned the reasons for these high attendance rates; they simply assumed that all families attending the centers wanted medical checkups and health education. As reasonable as that assumption is, we cannot discount other possible attractions, such as a chance to get into town to socialize and see friends; an opportunity to demonstrate the superior health of one's child; and the like. Whatever their motives, women who attended the centers were exposed to modern healthcare lessons.
[7]State Board of Health Assistant Public Health Nurse, District #7, "Narrative Report, November 1939," in *M&CH,* box 15, folder 10.

Wisconsin did not lack public health nurses. There were city nurses, county nurses, school nurses, Wisconsin anti-tuberculosis nurses, and Red Cross nurses. But there were many, especially rural, counties that had no public health nurses. In the midst of the Great Depression, county officials needed to be convinced to expend funds for nurses when, for example, road conditions presented a more immediate concern.[8]

THE MATERNAL AND CHILD HEALTH DEMONSTRATION NURSE PROGRAM

For years, the Wisconsin State Board of Health had tried to persuade counties to appoint public health nurses. At one period the legislature even appropriated $1,000 for each county to pay for a county nurse office. But few counties took advantage of this limited funding. With the Social Security Act of 1935, the Bureau of Maternal and Child Health obtained the funding for a more attractive package: the Maternal and Child Health Nurse Demonstration Program, through which the state would fund the salary and travel expenses for an MCH nurse, a demonstration nurse. The county paid only for office expenses and phone. The federal monies were earmarked for maternal and child health, but in insisting that "any family contacted through an expectant mother should have rendered by the nurse a generalized public health nursing service if the greatest benefit is to be derived from such as service," the bureau significantly expanded the scope of the program.[9] Accordingly, the demonstration nurse was a step toward a county public health nurse.

The MCH program placed its nurses in an awkward position. Through their work with mothers and children, these nurses were to demonstrate—to prove—the efficacy of public health nursing. What constituted proof? The program was proven when the county employed a county nurse. Thus, the demonstration nurses (all female at this time) needed to help their clients, curry favor with the local physicians (all male at this time), and convince local government officials (also primarily male at this time) and county residents that public health was a vital county responsibility. In the best of all circumstances, the demonstration nurse would simply slide into the position of county nurse. In some Wisconsin counties, that is what happened. In others, the demonstration nurse left and another nurse took her place as

---

[8]For more on public health nursing in the period, see Karen Buhler Wilkerson, *False Dawn: The Rise and Decline of Pubic Health Nursing, 1900–1930*, ed. Stuart Bruchey, *Garland Studies in Historical Demographic* (New York: Garland Publishing, 1989).
[9]Hunter, "Letter to Ed Jensen."

county nurse. In yet others, counties declined to appoint a county nurse and after 3 years or so, the county was left with no nurse. The conditions of each county were unique, but study of the efforts of one county, Barron County, will highlight the complicated roles that demonstration nurses played to effect the establishment and maintenance of a critical public health initiative.

PREVIOUS PUBLIC HEALTH EFFORTS IN BARRON COUNTY

Barron County had had at least four nurses between 1919 and 1922, but the position was abolished in the mid-1920s due to the economy.[10] In the late 1930s, the State Board of Health again sought to convince Barron's board of county supervisors to establish the position of county nurse. Board members were visited by the state's district health nurse, as well as the director of the Bureau of Public Health Nursing and the deputy health officer, but to no avail. The message was clear in 1939, as Margaret Brunner, the district health nurse, explained, "We planned to work for a county nurse this year, but were advised by the chairman of the finance committee not to appear before the board this year, as every budget was being cut." She saw hope for the future, however, noting that "next year the chairman of this committee stated he would work for a nurse, as he knew they needed a county nursing service."[11]

Disappointed, and acknowledging the county's acute need in fall 1939, the Bureau of Public Health Nursing arranged to send a nurse, Louise Steffen, to assist in the district health office. Steffen graduated from Mt. Sinai Hospital in Milwaukee, her hometown, and completed a certificate of public health nursing at Marquette University, also in Milwaukee.[12] By February 1940, Steffen was reassigned, establishing the county's first Maternal and Child Health Nurse Demonstration Program.[13] Dr. Amy Louise Hunter, chief of

---

[10]"Barron County," in *Wisconsin, Public Health Nursing Section, District health office correspondence, 1930–1972* (Madison, WI: Wisconsin State Historical Society box 3, folder: Barron County-Narrative Reports on.

[11]Margaret Brunner, "Annual Narrative Report for 1939," in *Wisconsin, Public Health Nursing Section, District advisory nurses' narrative reports, 1925–1968* (Madison, WI: Wisconsin State Historical Society) [hereafter referred to as *Pub Health Nursing. Ser. 908*], box 4, folder: Narrative Reports on District # 7 (May 31, 1953). Correspondence between the district office and the state office in Madison can be found in Louise Steffen, "Narrative Report for the Month of August, 1940," in *M&CH,* box 11, folder 10.

[12]Louise Steffen, "Letter to Cornelia Van Kooy, Dated November 20, 1939," in *Public Health Nursing, Series 905,* box 5, folder: 1936–1939, Social Security District 7.

[13]News clippings announcing Steffen's appointment are located in *M&CH,* box 11, folder 10.

Wisconsin's Bureau of Maternal & Child Health, was confident that with Steffen in the position, "the county will recognize the value of a service sufficiently to appoint a county nurse."[14]

LOUISE STEFFEN, RN, DEMONSTRATION NURSE

Steffen's reports to the bureau supported Hunter's optimism as she found, "On the whole, the attitude among the populace seems to be that this county should have had a county nurse long ago. I hope they will continue to think so and will, in the fall, still be of that mind." But, she also found local conditions unnerving:

> A great many of the families, [sic] have been referred to me by physicians, public welfare department, Farm Security Administration and lay people are on country roads that are very difficult to get to. I have had considerable difficulty and have not always been able to reach my destinations. The condition of the road is nothing new to the residents of the county, but is very new to me.[15]

And, she had to contend with physicians who complained that pregnant women did not come to see them early enough. The doctors recognized that county roads made visits difficult; that few women had available transportation to bring them into town; and that these poor women could not afford the fees that doctors charged for a home visit. But medical practitioners placed the burden of patient compliance on Steffen.[16]

These problems—unhelpful physicians, heavy workload, and inaccessible roads—continued to plague Steffen, though she assiduously built her caseload, contacted physicians, and waited for the roads to clear. Soon, the caseload grew such that, she cautioned,

> I possibly will have to limit the prenatal cases, eventually, to those referred to me by physicians. There is a tendency that only a small number of

---

[14]Amy Louise Hunter, "Letter to Dr. F. P. Daly, Dated January 27, 1940," in *Public Health Nursing, Series 905,* box 5, folder: District 7, 1940–1942.

[15]Louise Steffen, "Narrative Report for Month of February, 1940," in *M&CH,* box 11, folder 10.

[16]An important aspect of Steffen's work was identifying cases that needed the attention of a physician. I have found no evidence in the historical record that local physicians questioned this "diagnosing," in other words, practicing medicine. For more on the issue of differentiating nurses' clinical assessments and physicians' diagnostics, see Arlene Keeling, *Nursing and the Privilege of Prescription, 1893–2000* (Columbus, OH: Ohio State University Press, 2007).

> physicians would be served this way. There is also a tendency that the preschool caseload will get too large. I have been trying to limit it, but town chairmen and others get quite insistent about seeing cases. There have been referrals by several physicians, who at first were quite antagonistic, and now understand the service that is being given to the county.[17]

In convincing many people that her services were needed, Steffen was crushed by the tasks at hand. In her fourth month on the job, she reported that "More prenatals are being referred every day, more than I can get around to see."[18] By July, she grumbled that "A survey of the work thus far, [sic] was made, showing among other things that I have not been able to make neonatal visits on all cases seen during the prenatal period. The extent of the caseload does not allow it."[19] The tone of her monthly reports recounted the increasing tension she experienced between the press of her work with clients and the bureaucracy that work involved, her need to serve the bureau physicians when they held centers in the county, and her difficulties with local physicians. Some of the doctors welcomed her into their community, but at the same time swamped her with requests to see clients. Others disdained

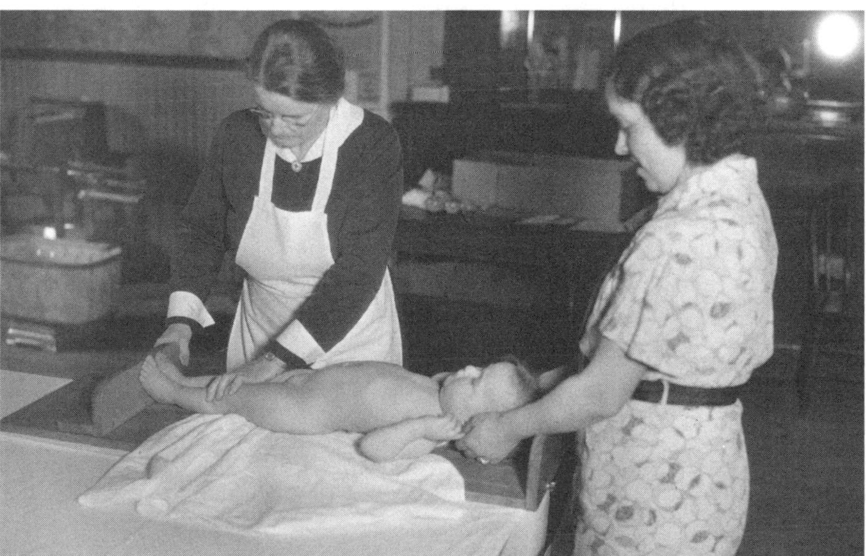

FIGURE 12.1 Unidentified mother helps an unidentified nurse examine her infant, ca. 1930s. *Reprinted with permission of the Wisconsin Historical Society.*

---

[17]Louise Steffen, "Narrative Report for Month of April, 1940," in *M&CH,* box 11, folder 10.
[18]Louise Steffen, "Narrative Report for the Month of May, 1940," in *M&CH,* box 11, folder 10.
[19]Louise Steffen, "Narrative Report for the Month of July, 1940," in *M&CH,* box 11, folder 10.

anything to do with the program and belittled her attempts. In a cryptic note, "Other things have occurred, but cannot be put to paper,"[20] she alluded to additional unspecified problems.

Steffen's employment review in the summer of 1940 substantiated many of her claims.[21] The state advisory nurse found Steffen "a conscientious, tireless worker" who "is dependable and sincere in her desire to 'sell nursing service' to Barron County." But her relationships with local physicians inhibited her efforts. Her caseload was concentrated in the west and southwest parts of the county, primarily because of "the excellent cooperation of the physician serving that area." Steffen needed to appear more throughout the county or "there may be criticism if too much time is given to Dr. Shima's patients." So, in answering requests from an interested physician, Steffen risked appearing to slight other areas of the county, even though the physicians there did not ask for her services. In addition, the MCH program required a local advisory council to assist the nurse in her efforts. At the end of July 1940 Steffen still lacked such a support network. The state advisory nurse explained that "Some attempt has been made to set up a lay advisory committee [Community Council] but, because of rivalries existing within the county, it has been difficult to decide on personnel." This rivalry was most likely the competition between the two leading towns in the county: Barron Township and Rice Lake, each of whom, for years, had vied to hold more child health centers than the other. Public health efforts, not surprisingly, were caught up in local politics.

Over the months, Steffen diligently educated the county about the importance of public health, though she worried that time spent in education distracted her from home visits. Still, in the month of August alone, "we have reached many people through child health centers and the Public Health exhibits at the County Fair. We had four child health centers, two of which had had a total attendance of 102. The other two were smaller, but were also large enough."[22] Eager to convert the demonstration program into a budgeted county position—the ultimate goal of the MCH program—Steffen was gratified in the fall of 1940 that "Various officials were contacted to get their reaction to the 'county nurse' situation. If they all stand by the things they say, we will have a county nurse here."[23] The next month she was less sanguine. Pleased that

---

[20]Ibid.

[21]This paragraph has been drawn from State Advisory Nurse, "Field Advisory Report [9/28/40]," in *M&CH,* box 11, folder 10; State Advisory Nurse, "Field Advisory Report [9/26/40]," in *M&CH,* box 11, folder 10.

[22]Steffen, "Narrative Report for the Month of August, 1940."

[23]Louise Steffen, "Narrative Report for the Month of September, 1940," in *M&CH,* box 11, folder 10.

"A great many people are convinced" of the need, she discovered "some of the town chairman [sic] and supervisors are *not* [stress in the original] convinced." Still, she remained optimistic because "We have been assured on many occasions that, 'of course, the county board must vote for a county nurse.'"[24]

BARRON COUNTY POLITICS AND PUBLIC HEALTH

The November 1940 County Board of Supervisors meeting surprised and disheartened Steffen:

> I never believed that the county board members would vote the county nurse question down, but after 5 days of waiting it was defeated . . . The county board chairman made a personal plea, but balancing the budget was uppermost in the minds of most of the members. One person, who promised active support for the issue and led us to believe that he could sway the county board, at the last minute said it would be impossible to balance the budget to include the necessary funds for a county nurse service.[25]

With the harsh light of politics, Steffen found that "my belief in the truthfulness and integrity of many individuals has been considerably shaken."[26] Her analysis was partly correct. The board defeated the motion on a vote of 31–19, with Supervisor C. D. Beckwith, chair of the finance committee, pleading budgetary constraint. There were, however, other objections. Supervisor Charles H. Sykes believed that a county nursing service would "set up a class discrimination." He wanted to submit a bill in the state legislature to place the service in the welfare department.[27] Since the service was intended for all families of Barron County, not just those on welfare, it would appear that Sykes did not understand the program, which suggests that more education was needed among the populace.

Steffen, though sorely disheartened, plunged ahead with renewed vigor. She reported that she was now a member of the local Community Council, the lay agency intended to support the demonstration nurse. This, she anticipated, "should be very helpful in furthering interest in the county nursing

---

[24]Louise Steffen, "Narrative Report for the Month of October, 1940," in *M&CH,* box 11, folder 10.
[25]Louise Steffen, "Narrative Report for the Month of November, 1940," in *M&CH,* box 11, folder 10.
[26]Ibid.
[27]"County Nurse Plan Refused by 31–19 Vote," *Rice Lake Chronotype*, November 20, 1940.

service."[28] Her activities promoting the county program increased, and she often related stories about the support she had in the community, particularly of those who took the board to task for its negative decision.[29] For example, in January 1941, she spoke with a local group that "promised to give personal cooperation and backing at the next county board meeting."[30]

In the spring, a "community-minded organization" held a charity dance that raised considerable funds. The Community Council "asked if [the nurse] would want the fund set up for her use." Aware of the political difficulties this could engender, Steffen suggested that instead the money be turned over to the county's Crippled Children's Fund, from which she could then draw. In addition, she could use the fund to provide glasses for needy children.[31] So too her caseload continued to grow. Though physicians referred only a few, more physicians were interested, especially when Steffen could provide a unique service, such as working out infant feeding problems.

Given the extent of her work with clients, with health centers, and the Community Council, Steffen continued to be baffled by the lack of support on the part of county supervisors, on the part of local physicians, even on the part of many members of the community. Why, she asked, does the county board more easily fund road repair than immunization projects; why is the county more interested in their livestock than their children's health? Chaffing under the pressure of her caseload and the "numerous storms and thawing weather [that made] travelling difficult," in March 1941 she was particularly eloquent about her concerns.

> The "county nurse" question comes up every day. Such a great deal is done in this county to perfect the health of the dairy herds, but what about the health problems among the people? Is it agreeable with the State Board of Health if a concentrated campaign is put on to put this question before the people. I realize that great care must be taken in the kind of material that is selected but many people do not know the health problems that exist in the county.[32]

There is no record of the board's response, and Steffen's monthly reports continued to note the same problems.

---

[28]Steffen, "Narrative Report for the Month of November, 1940."

[29]Louise Steffen, "Narrative Report for the Month of December 1940," in *M&CH,* box 11, folder 10.

[30]Louise Steffen, "Narrative Report of the Month of January, 1941," in *M&CH,* box 11, folder 10.

[31]Louise Steffen, "Narrative Report for the Month of April, 1941," in *M&CH,* box 11, folder 10.

[32]Louise Steffen, "Narrative Report for the Month of March 1941," in *M&CH,* box 11, folder 10.

STEFFEN'S LAST MONTHS IN BARRON COUNTY

For some unspecified reason, Steffen had a 3-month leave, July through September 1941, which resulted in unanticipated benefits. First, the nurse's office had been moved from a tiny office in the relief department to more spacious quarters on the second floor of the court house, which in Steffen's judgment "couldn't be any better." Second, and most important, her absence was "really missed by various organizations, physicians and families that have been previously visited." But the return was not without problems. In addition to handling a "great many new cases," a county board meeting was approaching.[33] With the position of county nurse again on the agenda, Steffen placed a report of her work before the board, something she had not done at the preceding meeting.

Steffen's two-page report was printed in full in the *Proceedings of the County Board of Supervisors*. Perhaps she was convinced that the board would not appropriate funds for a county nurse; perhaps she was frustrated with the numerous obstacles she faced, but for whatever reason, a scolding tone pervaded the report. She began "Because many people believe, and perhaps some of you too, that there is a county nurse in Barron County, I will briefly again [!] tell you just what kind of a public health nursing service there is here." A short explanation of the Maternal and Child Health Nurse Demonstration Program followed, listing the services she provided to pregnant women, new mothers, and young children and her involvement in health centers, and ending with "May I take this opportunity to thank the county officials, physicians, newspapers and the various county agencies for their interest and cooperation in making the nursing service more adequate."[34] "More adequate"? Not more successful, but "more adequate," a virtual slap in the face to the board for its inattention to the issue.

The board *Proceedings* did not note any discussion of the report, or even any response to it. The one-sentence in the local newspaper, "The report of Miss Louise Steffen, child and maternal health nurse, revealed wide activity during the last 17 months,"[35] was equally nonresponsive. As Steffen had feared, the board did not care to spend money on a county nurse position; rather, the "general sentiment seemed to be 'Why should we worry about something that we get free of charge now? Next year [when the MCH Program was due to expire] we will start worrying about it[sic].'"[36]

---

[33]Louise Steffen, "Narrative Report for Month of October, 1941," in *M&CH,* box 11, folder 10.
[34]*Proceedings of the County Board of Supervisors of Barron County* (Barron, WI: 1941), 111–112.
[35]"County Board," *Rice Lake Chronology*, November 19, 1941.
[36]Louise Steffen, "Narrative Report for the Month of November, 1941," in *M&CH,* box 11, folder 10.

Shortly thereafter, Steffen accepted a position in Milwaukee.[37] No reason was given for her resignation. Possibly her earlier 3-month leave indicated a medical or family emergency that required her to return to Milwaukee. Maybe she found Barron County and its politics and poverty too overwhelming. Conceivably she preferred city life to life in rural Wisconsin. Whatever the reason, Steffen left and the position remained open until January 1943 when Hazel A. Nordley reestablished the Maternal and Child Health Nurse Demonstration Program in Barron County for the remaining months of its term. Unlike Steffen, Nordley grew up in northern Wisconsin, in Superior. She graduated from St. Mary's Hospital Nursing School, also in Superior.[38]

HAZEL A. NORDLEY, RN, DEMONSTRATION NURSE

Nordley quickly threw herself into the work, sending letters to county supervisors and to physicians to alert them to resumption of the service. Within the first month, she was pleased to report that "quite a few cases have been referred so far." Though few had come from physicians, she was finding some physicians very glad to see her. Other doctors were uninterested, but, she optimistically related, "I hope in time they will all make use of the service." More positively, the chairman of the county board offered her the opportunity to report at the May board meeting.[39] Nordley's May report was politically more adept than Steffen's. She provided much more detail about her work, and especially stressed the importance of the nursing service in identifying cases early, citing an example to illustrate her point: a baby with a cleft palate and hair lip.

> The baby was very badly disfigured due to the hare lip, but at approximately 6 weeks of age was admitted to the Orthopedia Hospital for surgery with wonderful results. He wouldn't be recognized as the same baby. Had this surgery been delayed until the child was much older these good results would not have been possible.

Nordley gently urged the board to provide smallpox vaccination and diphtheria immunization, noting that "relatively few children" in the county were protected against these diseases, which were appearing throughout the state and especially in neighboring counties. Rather than reproach the board for

---

[37]Louise Steffen, "Narrative Report for the Month of December 1941," in *M&CH,* box 11, folder 10.

[38]Hazel A. Nordley, Registration, *Wisconsin Board of Nursing: Permanent Record Cards, Series 2675, reel 6* (Madison, WI: Wisconsin State Historical Society).

[39]Hazel A. Nordley, "Narrative Report for Month of January, 1943," in *M&CH,* box 11, folder 10.

its failures, she offered a solution to a potential problem: "How long it will be before [smallpox and diphtheria] strike here, we don't know. Wouldn't it be worth while [sic] to see that the youngsters are vaccinated and immunized before such a thing occurs." She pointed out that she could not visit the many tuberculosis cases in the county and other potential health problems that occurred outside the maternal/child family setting and solicited the help of the board to improve the health of the county by referring cases to her.[40]

How successful this more inclusive approach was compared with Steffen's reprimand is difficult to judge from this historical distance. Local newspapers did not carry many stories about the county nurse's question. Nordley herself discussed it very little in her monthly reports back to Madison, though in a fall report, she complained that people still thought of her as a "county nurse" whose duties were not limited to maternal and child health concerns. On a more positive note, she considered interactions with board members encouraging: "Any contacts I've had with board members have been satisfactory but just what they will do when it comes to a vote [in November], I don't know."[41]

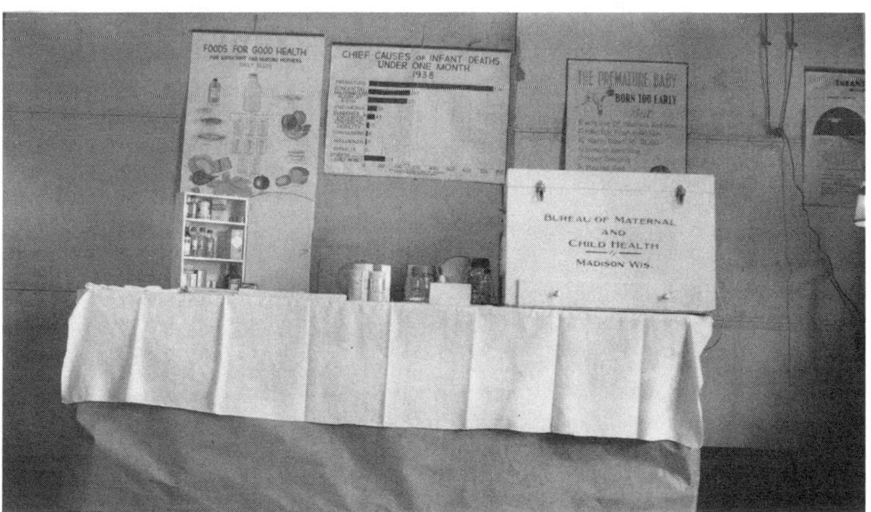

FIGURE 12.2 Exhibit produced by Louise Steffen for the Barron County Fair, Barron, Wisconsin, 1940. *Reprinted with permission of the Wisconsin Historical Society.*

[40]Hazel A. Nordley, "To the Honorable Members of the County Board of Supervisors of Barron County [May 1943]," a carbon copy of typescript is located in *M&CH,* box 11, folder 10.
[41]Hazel A. Nordley, "Narrative Report for Months of August and September [1943]," in *M&CH,* box 11, folder 10.

With the Maternal and Child Health Nurse Demonstration Program due to expire at the end of December 1943, the director of the Bureau of Public Health suggested "it would be advisable to get a complete report of the work accomplished by the nurses assigned to the demonstration program in time for the November County Board meeting and if possible, such a report should be mailed to each member of the County Board before he comes to the meeting, with a letter suggesting support for the employment of a county nurse."[42] Nordley's fall report employed the same strategies as her May one. She opened with a reminder that her work was restricted to mothers, children, and their families. Thus, "this demonstration service is really inadequate in a county, because it leaves so many health problems uncared for in homes that do not come under the above specifications."[43] Then, in providing the board with the cumulative statistics of the service's work from February 1940 to the present, she adroitly advanced the case for a county nurse and specified the benefits such as home visits, case follow-up, education of pregnant women and new mothers, and identification of communicable diseases, as well as health centers, in other words, the advantages of preventive medicine. She also made the case for a county nurse very concretely with an economic argument that might resonate more with the board.

> During the 10 year period 1930–1940 the total cost of sanatarium care for Barron County residents was $103,098.72. Much of this expense as well as suffering for the patient could be avoided if cases were found early and treated. Finding contacts and having them examined and treated when needed would do much toward accomplishing this goal.[44]

She concluded:

> It is felt that the demonstration program in Barron County has been a success but the drawback is that it does not cover a wide enough field. What is needed is a well planned, well organized, generalized public health nursing service for the entire county. One principle that governs all public health work is fundamental—to give the greatest protection to the greatest number of persons with the least expenditure.[45]

---

[42]Cornelia van Kooy, "Letter to Mrs. Vivian H. Werner, Advisory Nurse-District #7, Dated September 24, 1943," in *Public Health Nursing, Series 905,* box 5, folder: 1943–1945 District Sanitary #7.

[43]Hazel A. Nordley, "Report of Maternal & Child Health Demonstration Nurse," *Proceedings of the County Board of Supervisors of Barron County,* 1943, p. 24. A typescript copy of the report is located in *M&CH,* box 11, folder 10.

[44]Ibid., 30.

[45]Ibid., 31.

Nordley detailed the important contributions of the MCH program, contributions that could be significantly enlarged with a county nurse program, she reminded the board.

THE 1943 DECISION OF THE BARRON COUNTY BOARD

And, the board did appropriate funds for a county nurse. "Needless to say," Nordley explained in her monthly report,

> it was quite a surprise to get a unanimous vote now after the majority of them had voted against it for so many years. I hope by the end of the year they will be convinced that a public health nurse can do a valuable piece of work in a county, instead of feeling that she only makes additional expense by "ordering" glasses, tonsillectomies and so on for children in relief families.[46]

The silence of the historical record makes it difficult to determine exactly what led board members to change their long-standing opposition. Several hypotheses are likely. By 1943, the financial conditions in the county were slowly changing, improvements brought by the New Deal and the war economy. Perhaps earlier resistance had been primarily monetary and the new situation alleviated that concern. Then, too, as doctors and nurses were pulled into the war effort, fewer healthcare providers were left in the rural areas of the country. Between 1942 and 1945, Barron County lost nearly one-third of its physicians.[47] Maybe the paucity of practitioners impelled the board to recognize a growing need for assistance. In earlier years, local organizations had promised to petition the board on behalf of the county nurse office. Possibly they did so in 1943, and we simply have no documentation of their involvement. Conceivably the board members had finally come to realize that modern medicine, particularly public health, offered much to the county.

But, undoubtedly, Hazel A. Nordley, herself, was a major influence. It is not clear that Steffen would have been successful if she had stayed in Barron County. Her monthly reports documented her discomfort with the local conditions. Was it because she was moving from an urban area to a rural area?

---

[46]Hazel A. Nordley, "Narrative Report for Month of November, 1943," in *M&CH*, box 11, folder 10.

[47]A study of the Wisconsin Medical Society and the American Medical Association directories of the period reveal that in 1942 there were 26 physicians in Barron County, the majority in Barron township, and Rice Lake. By 1945, the number was down to 14—at least 4 of whom joined the armed forces. The location of the others is not known.

Was it because she was of German extraction and Barron County was dominated with Scandinavians? Nordley was from Superior, Wisconsin, a relatively small city; she was of Swedish heritage. The backgrounds and personalities of the two women may have made a difference. What we do know is that through her work with women and children, her reports, and her interactions with board members, Nordley provided the evidence needed to recognize the benefits of a county nurse and a public health office for the local families. Obviously, Nordley believed that her fall report convinced wavering board members to vote in the affirmative. That they supported Nordley is also apparent since she was appointed the first county nurse in Barron County, a position she held for many years.

CONCLUSION

The history of Barron County's experiences with the Maternal and Child Health Nurse Demonstration Program exemplifies the pivotal role that nurses had, and continue to have, in the development and implementation of public health policies. The statistical reports of Steffen and Nordley revealed that the health of infants and families improved with their services. But good works alone were not sufficient. Steffen and, most particularly, Nordley needed to make and made conscious efforts to educate the county about the necessity for public health. The successful establishment of the county nurse in Barron County represents the critical conjunction of public health education and education about public health. As the contemporary studies of the NFP demonstrate, a successful two-pronge strategy continues to be needed today in maintaining public health initiatives.

CHAPTER 13

The Visit: Nurse Practitioners and the Negotiation of Practice

Julie A. Fairman

INTRODUCTION

Nurse practitioners derive their power from their clinical practice. This idea assumes the presence and preferences of the patient, as practice does not occur without its target, and also the presence, actions, and thoughts of the nurse. Together, the nurse and the patient form a link that revolves around health and illness, the skills and knowledge of the nurse, and the needs and wants of the patient, who according to recent polls highly values this relationship.[1] Clinical practice, then, is shaped by more than functional and technical tasks, but also by the partnership created through individual and personal interactions during a patient visit.

Of course, the association between patient and nurse practitioner is also shaped by many other factors, such as the context of healthcare, place of practice, and the complexities of payment. And, nurse practitioners do not practice in a vacuum; the space where practice occurs is very crowded. One could argue that autonomous practice is in reality impossible to achieve—all providers are part of a larger system that includes public and private institutions, communities, and other providers. In particular, the relationship between nurses and physicians as they navigate the shifting boundaries of

[1]Karen Donelan, Peter Buerhaus, Catherine Desroches, Robert Dittus, and David Dutwin, "Public Perceptions of Nursing Careers: The Influence of the Media and Nursing Shortages," *Nursing Economics* 26, no. 3 (2008): 143–150, 165, http://www.medscape.com/viewarticle/576950 (accessed October 12, 2009).

clinical practice determines how patients will access the healthcare system, the services they will receive, who provides them, and how they will pay for them. All of these factors interact within the metaphorical and physical boundaries of "the visit."

This chapter will examine how nurse practitioner practice is negotiated in the constructed space of the visit, what happens within this space, and how the power of the space itself is constantly negotiated and assigned, leading to collaborative practice. The visit may be flexible and ever changing, with its boundaries morphing according to its purpose and place. The value of using the visit as a unit of analysis is that it is historically flexible and serves as a snapshot of how nurses' clinical practice changes over time and location. As such, it becomes a proxy for practice. The voices of early nurse practitioners in the 1970s will be used to illustrate how the structure of the visit formed and reformed as patients and practitioners tested and expanded practice boundaries, negotiated the practice space, and formulated new practice models. Nurse practitioners and physicians will be the focus of this analysis, as both professions struggled to serve patients and maintain their professional authority and identity.

THE VISIT

The visit can be conceptualized in many ways. Perhaps most traditionally it serves as the basic unit of provider–patient interaction, which typically occurs in a physical space, and is used to categorize provider reimbursement. For example, an appointment in a clinic or private office for wellness or illness care is a traditional measurement. In the 1970s, nurse practitioners encountered patients in clinics, emergency rooms, and doctors' offices (the outpatient arena will be the focus of the chapter), chiefly under the authority of physician colleagues. Today, the place of nurse practitioner practice is fluid; it has expanded to include almost any space where they interact with patients—drugstore clinics, big-box stores, churches, homes, and schools in addition to the more traditional places of public health and institutional clinics. But the unit of the "office visit" still defines provider payment, service volume, and workload.

The broadening venue is just one indication of nurse practitioners' growing facility with clinical negotiations.[2] Whereas nurse practitioners of the 1970s may have deliberately chosen practice sites that were on the margins,

---

[2]Collaboration is exemplified broadly in this paper by the daily practice relationship established between physicians, patients, and nurses, and the supporting context of the visit. See Judith Baggs and Madeline Schmitt, "Collaboration between Nurses and Physicians," *Image* 20 (1988): 145–149.

with supportive physicians and little institutional oversight, nurse practitioners today are in demand in very public venues. Another historical difference might be the way nurses entered into these practice sites. Early nurse practitioners in the 1970s many times enlarged their role from a position they already occupied as office and clinic nurses familiar with the physicians they worked for. Modern nurse practitioners are found not only in these settings, but also establish their own practices or are hired through corporate chains, hospitals, and community-based clinics that are nurse managed.

Another way to think about the visit is perhaps, more conceptually, as a space where practice boundaries are negotiated by providers and patients, and the foundation for power and authority is established. Practitioners talk about "seeing" a patient, using metaphorical language to describe both the physical aspects of the visit—to actually visualize (and perhaps charge) the patient—and to "see" their problems through the more abstract process of clinical examination and diagnosis. Traditionally, physicians controlled the clinical space occupied by patient and provider, setting the boundaries of where the visit could occur, what it encompassed, what was accomplished, and who could see the patient.

The visit was, on the surface, a tightly controlled space shaped and ordered by physicians and their professional organizations. This scenario is more complicated if the broader constructs of health and illness are acknowledged as shape shifters, as forces that over time have also defined the visit. Insurers, legislators, professional organizations, and the public are all stakeholders at the point of practice, crowding and jostling for the opportunity to shape interactions and services. Providers and patients must manage all of these interests, and their ability to do so is contingent on their ability to negotiate the political terrain of stakeholders into a coherent collaborative relationship.

In the early 1970s, as the nurse practitioner movement gained momentum, broader policy issues such as state professional practice acts, reimbursement rates, and organizational politics influenced the place and types of services nurse practitioners provided during the visit. Strict state practice acts that mandated immediate supervision ensured that nurse practitioners practiced near physicians. Alert and competition-fearing medical societies with their larger pool of resources and political influence monitored what nurse practitioners and their physician colleagues were doing, and spearheaded prosecution of practice act infringements.[3] And the refusal of most third-party insurers at least into the late 1970s to individually and fully reimburse nurse

---

[3]The Pennsylvania State Board of Medical Examiners and Licensure, minutes, 10/22/71, 1/6/72, 12/4/73, Office of the Commissioner of Professional and Occupational Affairs, Harrisburg, Pennsylvania.

practitioners for their services ensured and required them into forced relationships with physician colleagues.

But despite the influence of these broader forces, the individual negotiations between nurses, physicians, and patients were powerful shapers of practice at the point of care. It was here that negotiations defined both the metaphorical and physical visit, with nurses securing permission from physicians to engage patients, earning patients' trust, and gaining self-confidence to create collaborative and independent encounters so that patients could benefit from nursing practice. The act of a nurse practitioner entering into a negotiation with a physician reshaped practice from the start, establishing an environment where questioning of practice boundaries and practice expansion could safely occur. Negotiation set forward a foundation for establishing collaborative practice, and it is in this conceptual space that the physical and metaphorical idea of the visit was actualized, as both the functional and the intellectual process that encompassed mutual interactions and dialogue between the provider and the patient.

Negotiations shaped collaborative practice within the context of the visit, moving it across a continuum of abstractness as the boundaries of practice were explored, defined, and redefined. Practice was actualized and standardized by the structure of rules and protocols jointly developed by providers and patients during the visit. But the process was also quite fluid. Collaboration was preceded by a process of boundary shifting between individual nurses and physicians that both tested and established contested terrain, illuminated the importance of trust and respect, and provided a frame from which negotiated practice could proceed. These negotiations were embedded in contextual shifts in nursing and medical education and practice, gender, federal entitlement policies, and economics of the post–World War II society.

To understand the roots of contemporary practice negotiations leading to collaboration, its complexity, and how it was shaped within the context of the visit, we must first think about how doctors and nurses navigated and negotiated their work in the changing healthcare environment 40 years ago and what interacting with patients during the visit meant for them.

SETTING THE FOUNDATION FOR THE VISIT

Nurse practitioners and physicians in the early 1970s were influenced by a rapidly changing social and economic milieu that created the framework for modern healthcare and health policy. For example, in the 1960s Lyndon Johnson's Great Society entitlement programs such as Medicare and Medicaid expanded the number of people who could afford private physician care, but came during a critical period of shrinking numbers of primary care physicians and a general policy of deinstitutionalization of the chronic and mentally ill.[4] Although Model Cities programs, part of Great Society initiatives, supported community clinics in underserved areas, patients in poor urban and rural areas still suffered from a lack of access to basic health services because of a shortage of healthcare providers. In 1965, the President's Commission on Heart Disease, Cancer, and Stroke issued its report and targeted both medical research funding and prevention programs in communities. Regional medical programs, an outgrowth of the report and the public movement supporting the right to healthcare, began to target these diseases in rural communities. Additionally, there was a general movement by the public to have more control over healthcare decisions and to generally be more informed about their healthcare. Many social movements such as the Women's movement, the Civil Rights movement, and the Anti-War movement, and strong labor organizations asserting their right to strike created a sense of tension as conservative and liberal groups fought for their place in society. The Women's Health movement, just taking hold during this time, emboldened women to more closely examine and participate in their own healthcare, and nurse practitioners were seen as a preferable alternative to the paternalism found in medicine. Nursing became a career choice for some women in the movement who saw what nurses could accomplish and felt drawn to a women-provided type of care.[5] Additionally, both economic inflation and recession contributed to the instability and uncertainty felt by the nation.

Nursing and medical education and practice were not immune from the societal changes occurring during the 1960s and 1970s. Nursing education slowly moved into colleges and universities, where critical thinking and individualized care became new models of practice. The College of Nursing at University of Florida, Gainesville, headed by Dean Dorothy Smith exemplified the new spirit of theory-based practice and clinical expertise, opening up both the hospital and the clinic as specific sites for nurses to directly engage patients in expanded roles.[6] Medical practice and education were becoming more specialized as fewer students entered the less lucrative primary care and general medical arena and opted for higher paying specialties with practices in affluent suburban communities. Report after report issued by the American Medical Association (AMA) and

---

[4]For an overview of these changes see Julie A. Fairman, "Delegated by Default or Negotiated by Need: Physicians, Nurse Practitioners, and the Process of Clinical Thinking," *Medical Humanities Review* 13, no. 1 (Spring 1999): 38–58.
[5]Susan Reverby, personal communication, 2009.
[6]Julie Fairman, *Making Room in the Clinic: Nurse Practitioner and the Evolution of Modern Health Care* (New Brunswick, NJ: Rutgers University Press, 2008).

other medical groups, although applauding the high level of medical expertise and technology found in American hospitals and medical schools, decried the shortage of physicians in poor rural and urban areas and the shortage of medical technicians (as nurses and others were labeled). The reports targeted similar solutions of using nurses to ease the load of primary care physicians (instead of using nurses for clerical work) and advocated medical control over the training of technicians, foreshadowing the 1990s debate over registered care technicians.

Through the 1960s and 1970s, the federal government infused large amounts of funds into the healthcare system through the support of nurse and physician education programs via various manpower and nurse training acts. Many innovative programs emerged from this spirit of federal largesse and milieu of change. Both the graduate program to train nurse practitioners at the University of Colorado and the Physician Assistant Program at Duke University emerged in 1965. Moreover, many of these federal programs, such as Title 10, paid for the training and practice of nurse practitioners in rural and urban health clinics.[7] All of these changes provided the opportunity for creative nurses and physicians to develop working relationships that were entrepreneurial and ground breaking, and to engage in the kind of dialogue that redefined both the location and character of the visit.

NEGOTIATING CLINICAL PRACTICE DURING THE VISIT: NURSE PRACTITIONER STORIES

In the nurse practitioner–physician dyad, negotiations centered on nurse practitioners' right to access patients on a more independent level and practice an essential part of traditional medicine, the process or skill set of clinical thinking. In this chapter, clinical thinking encompasses the formalized skills, knowledge, and language that physicians traditionally used to organize and collect particular patient data (e.g., perform a physical examination, elicit patient symptoms, and given the symptoms, order diagnostic tests), create a diagnosis, formulate treatment options, prescribe treatment, and make decisions about prognosis.[8] The ability to use the language of clinical thinking, especially the politically loaded terms of diagnosis and prescription, was an

---

[7]Denise Geolot, "Federal Funding of Nurse Practitioner Education: Past, Present and Future," *Nurse Practitioner Forum* 1, no. 3 (December 1990): 159–162.
[8]Julie A. Fairman, "Delegated by Default or Negotiated by Need: Physicians, Nurse Practitioners, and the Process of Clinical Thinking," *Medical Humanities Review* 13, no. 1 (1999): 38–58; Barbara Bates, *A Guide to Physical Examination and History Taking*, 6th ed. (Philadelphia, PA: J.B. Lippincott, 1995), 635–648.

important part of the unacknowledged process of negotiating cultural authority and intellectual space. The authority to use the language inherent in the clinical thinking process bestowed a sense of legitimacy, a sharing of the conceptual universe of medicine. The linguistics of medicine within this universe became a highly contested intellectual space that had implications for nurse practitioner identity and status as socially accepted healthcare providers.

The negotiations leading to collaborative practice centered on clinical thinking because intellectual and practical discussions concerning patient care problems centered on this skill and its language. Clinical thinking was most intense and the opportunity for dialogue and problem solving most likely at the bedside or in the exam room, between individual nurses, physicians, and patients. At the point of care, the negotiations were continuous, and involved informal and sometimes tacit social interactions framed by the personalities of the individual doctors, nurses, and patients.[9]

Initially, close proximity of practitioners and receptivity of both nurse practitioners and doctors to listen and to dialogue was key. One nurse practitioner noted, "Initially we had to always have a physician on site for instance, when we were doing clinical work. And I didn't resent that. Actually, I needed the backup."[10] But, as the negotiations progressed and trust was established on both sides, availability rather than close physical proximity was required. "I was seeing the patients [in rural Western Pennsylvania] with the physicians on call for me in Pittsburgh," one nurse noted, "You and I both know they're not coming out here. So they were available to me on the phone...."[11] In this way, the space of the visit became more flexible and fluid, expanding from physical proximity and architectural structures to broader virtual space defined by the technology and communication.

Many early nurse practitioners also describe examples that illustrate physicians' difficulty relinquishing the symbolic accoutrements of the visit. Even when the competency of the nurse practitioner was unquestioned, physicians sometimes repeated procedures such as taking the patient's blood pressure or pulse. These repetitive, ritualistic actions had less to do with lack of trust than physicians' need to maintain their personal connection and perhaps, their relevancy with patients. These were skills that had long been taken over by nurses in general, but generated new meanings and power for physicians struggling to adjust to changing clinical contours of the visit.

Amorphous negotiations, like the establishment of trust through knowledge trades, were essential processes for defining the clinical space

---

[9]Fairman, "Delegated by Default...."

[10]CJ, oral history interview by M. J. Murphy, September 20, 1997, telephone interview.

[11]BR, oral history interview by M. J. Murphy, September 18, 1997, telephone interview.

of collaborative practice. "In the beginning he was real gentle in letting me do things. Don't even make a referral without him, don't do this. Don't do that. But soon he [knew] you well enough.... It is a situation you have to go through with each physician, and I had a lot of them, and we probably taught them a lot of their basic people skills they [didn't] learn in their training."[12] Although the status of the knowledge trade might have been perceived by the professions as unequal, the medical skill holding greater perceived status over the communicative skills, each nurse practitioner and physician contributed to the relationship, and each learned from the other.[13]

Negotiations were supported by the mutual dependency of medical and nursing professionals as they struggled together to provide healthcare for their clients and meaningful work for themselves. In fact, and perhaps most germane to this argument, negotiations and the collaboration they led to were not mandated "from above" by the edicts of national organizations such as the AMA or the American Nurses' Association (ANA), or educational institutions. In fact, neither the AMA nor the ANA were initially supportive of the concept of the nurse practitioner.[14] Negotiation and collaboration happened in a seemingly disconnected way in many different places, and only later came together as a movement. "This all [nurse practitioners working with physicians] occurred because [the] physicians knew us and felt that we had good judgment—we had worked with them before...."[15] The process was personal, individualistic, rather than institutional, and served the needs of the triad of both practitioners and patients.

Although imbalances in power and skill status existed between the nurse and physician negotiators, and each party may have held different perspectives of how negotiations proceeded or how the patient visit would be constructed, incongruent power and perspective did not prevent the process from occurring because both physicians and nurses obtained what they needed or wanted.[16] Among other things, physicians received help in their busy practices and the freedom to pursue more interesting cases by teaching nurses to perform various parts (e.g., physical examination, history taking, decision making based on the data collected) of the clinical thinking process. "Very quickly," one nurse explained, "I got to do all of the stuff he didn't want to do, which was the

---

[12]FD, oral history interview by M. J. Murphy, September 24, 1997, telephone interview.

[13]Linda Schiebinger, *Has Feminism Changed Science?* (Cambridge, MA: Harvard University Press, 1999).

[14]Natalie Holt, "Confusion's Masterpiece: The Development of the Physician Assistant Profession," *Bulletin of the History of Medicine* 72, no. 2 (Summer 1998): 246–278.

[15]CJ, oral history interview.

[16]Julie Fairman, "Watchful Vigilance: Nursing Care, Technology, and the Development of Intensive Care Units," *Nursing Research* 41 (January/February 1992): 56–60.

physicals, which was fine."[17] She added, "...he [the physicians] taught us to do things that needed to be done when he couldn't get there, like suture lacerations.... We got good at it.... Our insurance carrier came out and said "don't do that," but he wanted us to do everything we could to help him....[18] Another nurse added, "He [the physician] was in one clinic 1 day, and another clinic another day. He had a private practice too. But he was always available by phone and always responded immediately."[19]

Participating nurses, in turn, agreed to the instruction and were eager to take on skills traditionally performed by medical professionals. "So I was really with him [the physician] like two and a half days and really learned an awful lot from him. He was very patient and like I said, he didn't have a problem with nurses learning to do this and he really taught. And I really learned to take care of a lot of the abnormal patients. Before I quit he was already teaching me how to do fertility things, which was pretty unheard of back then."[20] Nurses received the benefits of status linked to the skills, and the ability to practice in new and more meaningful ways that corresponded with their experience and education. "I didn't have to rely on what the physicians said. I had my parameters and I could treat a patient within them. I had my own decision making. I was a lot more independent, autonomous and it did a lot to help me realize that hey, I can do this, I'm not dumb. I can do this, and then as I learned more and more, I really was able to do the things for patients that I had always wanted to do for years and had to wait for a physician to agree. I could take care of the problems I saw. It relieved frustration."[21]

When nurse practitioners went outside familiar territory of already established visit parameters or entered into new relationships, the importance of the local, personal character of their negotiations was sometimes quickly made apparent. At the University of Rochester, Rochester, NY, early nurse practitioner Joan Lynaugh and her nurse and physician colleagues held a "clandestine clinic," where they could practice and learn together without arousing the suspicions of others who did not believe in expanded nursing practice.[22] A nurse from another setting explained, "I almost never saw [another] physician. It [contact with physicians] was almost always on the phone. There was more antagonism. 'An NP? What is that, what did you do? Who did the exam? You did the exam? Well, was there a doctor there?"[23] Outside of the frame of

---

[17]FD, oral history interview.
[18]Ibid.
[19]BR, oral history interview.
[20]Ibid.
[21]Ibid.
[22]Fairman, *Making Room in the Clinic.*
[23]CJ, oral history interview.

individual practices, nurses and doctors renegotiated the parameters of collaborative relationships and the parameters of the visit one, by one, by one. One nurse astutely described this individualist approach, "Any of my independent jobs, I went in with a physician who had never worked with an NP before and so I always started out very, very slowly, very cautiously. [I] would start out with, 'these are the things I can do, but you tell me what you want me to do.' And generally started out pretty restrictive. Self-restrictive because I wanted them to feel comfortable with my decision making and I wanted them to feel comfortable with how I did things and then slowly show them that I knew how to do some other things and that I would be glad to do it. You know, tell them that this woman has a big mass on the right side, it's pretty tender, I think we need to get an ultrasound. Is that what you want me to do?' And then, pretty soon, it was just—'Oh, you didn't need to call, just go ahead and do that.'"[24]

Negotiation of clinical space was a time-intensive, and sometimes painful, process. As this same nurse noted, "There were times when I would come home and say to my husband, 'Do I have holes in my head? Why am I doing this again?'" But, the negotiation process led to a mutually beneficial clinical practice, as the following nurse practitioner noted. "Although I was in the community, I was not working with any physicians from the community because the physician that worked in the clinic was from another town. So recognizing that we had patients that lived in this town, we felt the need to refer them, if they needed additional help, to a physician in the vicinity. So it was kind of hard getting those physicians to not grumble and growl, and to take you serious, recognize that you were doing something worthwhile and that you were not stupid." She went on, "But then as we were there longer and longer, and that when we sent a patient to them, that patient did in fact have an accurate diagnosis, had been treated well, things sort of settled down."[25]

In turn, nurse practitioners also had to trust that their physician colleagues would not expect or force them to go beyond mutually established boundaries. "I just trusted the physician I was working with that what he told me to do was ethical, proper, and legal . . ."[26] Of course, in the absence of concrete rules, individual creativity and needs held sway. Although each individual's state practice laws, and later, federal regulations should have served as a guide, within the framework of individual negotiations between nurse practitioners and physicians, there was room for contingency and flexibility, as the state regulations were sometimes vague. For example, in Pennsylvania, by 1977 both the State Board of Nursing and the State Board of Medical Education and

---

[24]BR, oral history interview.

[25]Ibid.

[26]FD, oral history interview.

Licensure regulations (in Pennsylvania, nurse practitioners were jointly promulgated) allowed that a nurse practitioner, "once qualified, could perform acts of medical diagnosis or prescription of medical, therapeutic or corrective measures *in collaboration with* and under the direction of a licensed physician...."[27] Collaboration was never defined in the state regulations although the acts of medical diagnosis and prescription were generally noted.

Distrust, lack of information, or personality incompatibility obstructed the negotiation process and made the visit a contested space. Collaborative practice could not be supported when the nurse practitioner and physician were unable to construct clear, mutually agreeable boundaries. Then, nurses and physicians working together resembled toddlers at parallel play rather than a more sophisticated intellectual and interactive practice. In one example, a newly graduated nurse practitioner was hired by a group of physicians to work in a North Philadelphia pediatric clinic that had received funding from the Models City program. She described the difficulty—"They [the physicians] weren't familiar with it [the nurse practitioner role]. They had gotten HEW funding to hire such a person. They had no clue, and I had almost no clue myself. I had a little more information than they did, but I was kind of looking for somebody to help me implement the thing, and they were like kinda filling a position because the government said 'hire such a person and pay them X salary. So it wasn't really clear what I was to do."[28] Although the lack of defined roles could have been quite liberating, nurse practitioners in their first job post-training wanted and needed new physician colleagues to understand their ability to contribute to the practice and to support them during their initial work experience.

The fledgling nurse practitioners found themselves in new situations where they were uncertain and untrusting of their own abilities, thus the trust embodied by physician colleague support was an extremely important ingredient in the negotiation process and construction of the visit. If they could not trust their physician colleagues to back them up when problems arose, collaborative practice was insupportable. "I let them know in the beginning that this was my first job and what I would need is a lot of checking things out with them, them becoming familiar with what I knew, learning from them because this was my first job. [But that] fell on deaf ears. They didn't seem to quite understand that it wasn't OK just to go to lunch if I had a patient with a 104 temp who possibly had meningitis. I would have to go find them in the lunchroom. They'd forget to turn their pagers on.... I didn't know whether they thought I could do it or if they just weren't on top of things."[29]

[27]*Pennsylvania Bulletin* 7(30); Saturday 23 July, 1977: 2061, 2063.
[28]DP, oral history interview.
[29]Ibid.

Without establishment of trust, and the lack of substantive negotiations, the nurse practitioners felt isolated, and their unique contributions to the care of patients in the clinic or practice went unacknowledged or invisible. Patient care may not have been compromised at its most basic level, but the potential for expanded services may have been limited. The nurse continued, "I don't have any good memory of them [the physicians] being very informative, I don't know if it just wasn't a great fit, but they sort of left me on my own. They didn't want to seem to make it fit. To find more of a support group, I used to go up to St. Christopher's. There were NPs up there I could hang with.... I could work with those nurses and...discuss common concerns that we had in clinical practice, what we were doing, how we were sorting thing out. It was useful."[30]

Seeking out other sources of validation and support helped nurse practitioners during their negotiations of the visit boundaries with physician colleagues. These sources ranged from the nurse practitioners support group described by the previous nurse to support from a particular patient group. A nurse practitioner working in the same practice since 1974 noted a familiar duality early on in her practice. "I was not the first NP in the practice...so it was already geared for NPs. It was harder in the hospital. We used to go on nursery rounds to convince them [hospital residents and other physicians]."[31] The nurse continued, "Now,...the nurses are so happy we're there. They think kids get better care on weekends and every baby gets examined. Every mother can see we are doing this. They always feel issues get dealt with more comprehensively when the NPs are there. So it's a full 180 from not having any backup to completely having a fan club."[32]

VISITING THE PRESENT

The willingness of both nurses and physicians to negotiate collaborative relationships is one infused with both continuity and change, depending upon the location, setting, time period, and the individual nurse–physician participants. The increasing complexity of patients, especially the chronically ill and older adults, and the intricacies of their treatments created a modern environment where negotiated collaborative practice is a necessity for physicians and nurses. Modern practice has become too complex, fragmented, emotionally charged, and intensely personal. It enfolds the social and personal relationships

---

[30]Ibid.
[31]BMC, oral history interview by M. J. Murphy, October 23, 1997, Philadelphia, PA.
[32]Ibid.

necessary for the provision of healthcare, and is part of the foundation upon which modern healthcare is defined. Because of the personal nature of this important social interaction within a particular contextual space, collaboration has proven difficult to establish by fiat, legislate, and sustain on a large scale. It is more commonly mandated as supervision clauses in state practice acts (e.g., one physician can supervise or develop collaborative practice agreements with a certain number of nurse practitioners), although these types of structures fail to encompass the relationship aspect necessary for negotiated collaborative practice.

In October 2009 the AMA released a series of 10 modules designed as advocacy tools for their members at the state level to educate legislators and the public about the dangers of practice boundary expansion of "limited license practitioners," including optometrists, audiologists, and nurse practitioners.[33] Although the term limited-license practitioners has been used for many years, the AMA's document reintroduced this negative language into the public domain at a very visible level, with possible implications for the way nurse practitioners and physicians negotiate the contours of the visit. The use of the language is a political maneuver intended to create a feeling of doubt in the public's perception of nurse practitioners in particular, and instill a sense of inadequate care. Its use suggests the threat providers such as nurse practitioners pose to the AMA at a time of great uncertainty in healthcare reform debates over who should provide healthcare to the American public. The providers addressed by the AMA modules present the greatest potential for expanded practice and medical authority during a time when shortages in physician supply threaten medicine's hold on patient care. In response to the physician shortage, the AMA realistically acknowledges in the modules the importance of team work and negotiation in clinical practice, but it remains mired in the same rhetoric it has used for decades: Patient safety is threatened by practice boundary expansion of nurse practitioners when negotiations go too far, despite decades of evidence to the contrary. Even the process of a comprehensive physical examination has been challenged by the AMA, the House of Delegates reaffirming in June 2009 that the function should be limited to physicians (both MDs and DOs) or under the direct supervision of physicians.[34]

---

[33]American Medical Association, *AMA Scope of Practice Data Sets: Nurse Practitioners* (Chicago, IL: AMA, October 2009).

[34]American Medical Association, House of Delegates, "Report of Reference Committee B, Resolution 235, Performance of a History and Physical by Non-Physicians," June, 2009, http://www.ama-assn.org/ama1/pub/upload/mm/475/a-09-ref-comm-b-annotated.pdf (accessed December 10, 2009).

At the national level, the AMA modules elicited a strong response by nurse practitioner organizations.[35] But, at the local level, during the visit, there appears to be little recognition or influence. Similar to the practice of early nurse practitioners, establishing the parameters of the visit remains a complex and individually negotiated process, but with different contextual factors across time and place. Nurse practitioners have become normative providers for many patients, and there is little public sentiment for changing the parameters of their relationships. As the oral narratives of the nurse practitioners suggest, the ability of individual practitioners to negotiate and construct functional and intellectual boundaries—the confines of the visit—is influenced more by the social environment and individual personality of the providers and patients than explicit directives from professional organizations or policy. In many ways, the collaborative process is still very much a social construction determined by contextual factors.

The area of practice shared by nurses and physicians within the confines of the visit is fluid and constantly changing, in part due to the complex and equally malleable societal perceptions of healthcare, technology, gender, and economics. Granted, the space of the visit is more than the acknowledgment of shared skill sets. It is an intellectual as well as a functional space that involves the negotiation of the skill set and the establishment of the rules of patient and provider engagement to most effectively devise solutions to patient problems. As practitioners know, creating a conducive and effective intellectual and clinical space for patient care is difficult to legislate, and even more difficult to negotiate on a large scale. Both parties in the relationship must be intellectually and philosophically compatible to see through the mire of healthcare politics and to the patient problems that await solution. As these narratives suggest, what happens within the confines of the visit, now construed in modern health reform discussions as more comprehensive and continuous than a singular point in time, is a very personal process that occurs on a foundation of trust and respect, and even the passage of time cannot remove the inherent intimacy nor potential power of the concept.

ACKNOWLEDGMENTS

This chapter is a revision of an earlier paper published in *Nursing History Review:* "The Roots of Collaborative Practice: Nurse Practitioner Pioneer Stories," 10 (2002): 159–174. The original work was supported by Sigma Theta Tau, Xi chapter and the Pew Charitable Trusts. The revision is supported by the Robert Wood Johnson Foundation Investigator in Health Policy Fellowship. The author thanks M. J. Murphy, research assistant, for her help on this project.

---

[35]Nursing Organizations to Michael Maves, December 8, 2009, http://www.aanp.org/AANPCMS2/publicpages/AMANPModuleLtr120809.pdf (accessed December 12, 2009).

CHAPTER 14

Nursing the Borderlands of Life: Hospice and the Politics of Health Care Reform

Joy Buck

INTRODUCTION

Kathy was 46 when she had her first heart attack, failed bypass surgery, and was permanently disabled due to a stroke. Before the fateful day when she collapsed at work, she had worked her way through nursing school and finally received her registered nursing licensure when she was 44. She then worked two jobs so she could afford to buy a house. Rather than realizing this dream, her savings were depleted as she struggled to pay her escalating medical debts. When she could no longer pay the bills, the collectors from the hospital where she used to work repossessed her car. As her health continued to decline, the nurses she once worked with distanced themselves. As they did, her identity as a colleague eroded and she came to feel as though she was "just a bunch of pills down the hall."[1] Exhaustion was a constant companion and despite having continuous oxygen, even the slightest activity winded her. Even reading, her one last pleasure, was taken away as her eyesight failed due to diabetic retinopathy. When she was finally admitted

[1]Anonymous, interview by author, June 2, 2009. The interview was done as part of a larger research project and permission was given to use the participant's story. Identifying information is not provided by request.

to a hospice program she was 54 and felt like a hostage, tethered to a trailer that was crumbling beneath her feet. Had she been referred to hospice earlier, the social worker could have referred her to another program to help pay her medical bills so she would not have lost her car. The nurses could have helped her manage her progressive physical symptoms, coordinate her care, and be available around the clock, 7 days a week, to help prevent unnecessary hospitalizations. As importantly, she could have gone on many more outings with her favorite volunteer who helped her regain her sense of humor and zest for life. It is not clear why she was not referred to hospice earlier—according to Medicare guidelines, she was "medically eligible" for services for at least 2 years before the cardiologist finally referred her. Perhaps he was reluctant to discuss her poor prognosis, did not understand the hospice eligibility criteria for people with noncancer diagnoses or did not realize how much she was in need of supportive services. Regardless of the reason, Kathy suffered needlessly as did her family as they helplessly watched her slowly wither away.

Kathy is just one of many Americans with progressive chronic illnesses who experience debilitating symptoms such as dyspnea, profound fatigue, and pain for several years before they die. They too might benefit from many of the types of services that hospice and palliative care promises. Yet, they rarely receive more than basic medical services that are often poorly coordinated and organized in a fashion that reinforces a false dichotomy between care for the "living" and care for the "dying." In large part, this is due to the way that healthcare is financed in the United States with regulations that aim to balance access to necessary services while controlling costs.

For better or worse, the politics of health policy shape almost every aspect of the American healthcare system and such is the case with hospice. The hospice philosophy of care was introduced to Americans in the 1970s as a necessary healthcare reform. Hospice advocates challenged many societal boundaries and assumptions about the appropriate care for the terminally ill. Yet, almost 30 years after hospice became an entitlement under the Medicare program, legislators continue to grapple with how to configure and finance healthcare for more than 90 million American adults with one or more chronic diseases.[2] Recent healthcare reform efforts have called for additional measures, such as "advance care planning" between health professionals

---

[2]John Wennberg, Elliott Fisher, David Goodman, and Jonathan Skinner, *Tracking the Care of Patients with Severe Chronic Illness: The Dartmouth Atlas of Health Care 2008, Executive Summary* (Lebanon, NH: The Dartmouth Institute for Health Policy and Clinical Practice, 2008).

and patients.[3] These proposed policy solutions are based on the premise that if people with progressive debilitating illnesses were fully informed, they would choose to enter hospice programs sooner rather than undergo aggressive therapies that may or may not be effective. Critics, however, contend that the advance directives provision will establish "death squads" who will "pull the plug on grandma." These charges are strikingly similar to the value-laden and emotionally charged rhetoric used by hospice critics during the 1970s. Then, hospices were called "death houses" where terminally ill patients and the disabled were given "dangerous narcotics," taught how to kill themselves, or refused treatment and sent on a "one way escalator toward death."[4] Why is it, then, that despite all the strides brought about by the hospice movement that the promise and possibilities of hospice remain so elusive? This chapter seeks to answer that question and by illuminating the past, to offer insight to help guide current and future palliative care initiatives.[5]

RIGHTS OF PASSAGE

The manner and location of care for the dying changed dramatically during the twentieth century. During the first half of the century, care for the dying was firmly within the domain of home, family, and religion. Family members, primarily women, would care for the dying person and prepare the body for burial when they died. For those with financial means, private nurses were hired to assist. Those without family or the means to pay for care in hospitals were sent to almshouses or asylums until they died.[6] In some circumstances, they were cared for in specialized homes for the dying that were founded by

---

[3]*America's Affordable Health Choices Act*, House of Representatives (Washington, DC, 2009), http://www.kff.org/healthreform/upload/housebill_final.pdf.

[4]No author, *Rocky's Do-It-Yourself Death,* New Solidarity, 1976, VII(43): 2.

[5]Joy Buck, "Reweaving a Tapestry of Care: Religion, Nursing, and the Meaning of Hospice, 1945–1978," *Nursing History Review* 15 (2007): 113–145; Joy Buck, "Home Hospice versus Home Health: Cooperation, Competition, and Cooptation," *Nursing History Review* 12 (2004): 25–46.

[6]Karen Buhler-Wilkerson, *No Place Like Home: A History of Nursing & Home Care in the United States* (Baltimore, MD: The Johns Hopkins University Press, 2001); Susan Smith and Dawn Nickels, "From Home to Hospital: Parallels in Birthing and Dying in Twentieth-Century Canada," *Canadian Bulletin of Medical History* 16, no. 1 (1999): 49–64.

religious groups from a variety of Christian and Jewish faith traditions.[7] This changed as federal legislation funded programs to expand the development of hospitals, support nursing and medical education, and advance medical science and technology. The resultant increase in the number of hospital beds and capacity for "life saving" was also due to larger societal trends such as population mobility, the transference of the extended family to the nuclear family, and women's work outside the home. By the end of the 1950s, more than 61% of deaths occurred in hospital.[8] The post–World War II rise in academic medical centers and the curative milieu within them had enormous implications in the social meaning of death and dying.

During the 1960s, research funded by the United States Public Health Service Division of Nursing documented the stark realities of institutionalized dying: Pain control was virtually nonexistent, and terminally ill cancer patients frequently died in a room at the end of the hall, in exquisite pain and alone.[9] Too often, the needs of patients and their families gave way to institutional and professional emphasis on medical knowledge, technology, and cost efficiency.[10]

While the medical mainstream remained relatively silent about these issues, many nurses and clergy did not. Nursing education began to focus on alternative approaches to care, ethical and spiritual issues related to death and dying, and research as a means to improve clinical practice.[11] The emergence of the discipline of pastoral counseling and hospital chaplains in academic medical centers helped reintroduce faith as an important element of care for hospitalized patients. Social movements outside the walls of medical institutions began to clamor for the reform of care provided within its walls. The civil and women's rights, death with dignity, and consumer movements laid a foundation for a growing public discourse about the quality of life, patients'

---

[7]Claire Humphreys, "Waiting for the Last Summons: The Establishment of the First Hospices in England 1878–1914," *Mortality* 6, no. 2 (2001): 146–166; Buck, "Reweaving a Tapestry of Care," 113–145.

[8]Monroe Lerner, "Where, Why, and When People Die," in *The Dying Patients*, eds. Orville G. Brim, Howard E. Freeman, Sol Levine, and Norman A. Scotch (New York: Russell Sage Foundation, 1970), 1–15.

[9]Barney G. Glaser and Anselm Strauss, *Time for Dying* (Chicago, IL: Aldine Press, 1968); Glaser and Strauss, *Awareness of Dying* (Chicago, IL: Aldine Publishing Company, 1965); David Sudnow, *Passing On: The Social Organization of Dying* (New Jersey: Prentice-Hall, 1967); Jeanne Quint, *The Nurse and the Dying Patient* (New York: The Macmillan Company, 1967).

[10]Eric Cassel, in *Death Inside Out: The Hastings Center Report*, ed. Peter Steinfels and Robert Veatch (New York: Harper and Row, 1974).

[11]Vicent Mor, David Greer, and Robert Kastenbaum, *The Hospice Experiment* (Baltimore, MD: The Johns Hopkins University Press, 1988).

rights, and the place of informed consent in the medical system.[12] Stories of how cancer patients suffered while undergoing aggressive curative treatment were widely publicized in the popular press. Despite the promise of curative medicine, many began to wonder if the quest for cure was worth the human toll in suffering.[13] It was within this context that the American hospice movement was born and British physician Dame Cicely Saunders emerged as one of its charismatic leaders.[14]

Conception and Birth of the American Hospice Movement

The modern hospice concept was first introduced to American health professionals in 1963 when Cicely Saunders made the first of many trips to North America.[15] During this first visit, Saunders spent 6 weeks traveling and lecturing about her work and research at St. Joseph's Hospice in London. She shared stories about patients who arrived at St. Joseph's expressing feelings of guilt and failure; some were at the brink of suicide due to unrelenting pain. She showed images of these patients as she spoke about the rejection many of them felt. In the words of a woman with breast cancer: "I knew I needed attention. They [previous hospital] never asked me back. They didn't see me, I didn't have any treatment, no pills or medicine or anything. I was so ill. When I came here everywhere I was in agony."[16] Saunders' charismatic speaking style and passion for hospice care resonated with a small but growing cadre of idealistic health professionals who would put hospice forth as the antidote for institutionalized

---

[12]See for example, Hugh Heclo, "The Sixties False Dawn: Awakenings, Movements, & Postmodern Decision Making," in *Integrating the Sixties: The Origins, Structure, and Legitimacy of Public Policy in a Turbulent Decade*, ed. Brian Balogh (University Park, PA: Pennsylvania University Press, 1996); James T. Patterson, "A Great Society and the Rise of Rights-Consciousness," in *Grand Expectations: The United States, 1945–1974* (New York: Oxford University Press, 1996), 562–593; W. J. Rorabaugh, "Challenging Authority, Seeking Community, & Empowerment in the New Left, Black Power, & Feminism," in *Integrating the Sixties*, ed. Brain Balogh, 106–143.

[13]Elisabeth Kubler-Ross, *On Death and Dying* (New York: Macmillan House, 1969); D. Gill, *Quest: The Life of Elisabeth Kubler-Ross* (New York: Harper and Row, 1988).

[14]Buck, "Reweaving a Tapestry of Care."

[15]Saunders' commitment to the care of terminally ill cancer patients began when she was working as a nurse at St. Luke's Hospice. She had to leave nursing for medical reasons, went on to train as a medical almoner (social worker), and then went on to medical training with the expressed purpose of reforming medical care for cancer patients.

[16]Cicely Saunders, *The Moment of Truth—Some Aspects of Care of the Dying Patient*, Presented at the Yale School of Nursing, April 28, 1966, Cicely Saunders Papers Hospice History Project, box 57, 3 (hereinafter CSPHHP).

dying in America. One of these professionals was Florence Wald, an American nurse who was then dean of the Yale School of Nursing.

For Florence Wald, Saunders's 1963 talk to the Yale University School of Nursing proved to be providential. A self-identified idealist, Wald was a leading advocate for major reforms in nursing education and the clinical role of the nurse.[17] She was dismayed by the growing trend in medicine to focus on cure and technology rather than on people. Frustrated clinical faculty and students often complained to her about physicians who refused to respond to patients' queries such as "What's wrong with me?" and "Am I going to get better?" When the nurses suggested that they might speak to the patients if the physicians were uncomfortable, they were met with: "If you're going to talk about this, I'm going to see that you're not allowed to see the patient anymore."[18] Saunders's depictions of hospice and the centrality of nursing within it was exactly the framework that Wald believed was necessary to spark significant reforms in nursing practice. Hospice offered the possibility of nurses and physicians to work together as equals in making decisions about patient care. Over the next several years, correspondence between Wald, Saunders, and a growing group of scholars and clinicians who shared a common commitment to reforming care for the dying proliferated. The free exchange of ideas and research created a connectedness and synergy between them that served as the catalyst that ignited and fueled the American hospice movement.[19]

By 1966, the year that Saunders returned to Yale as the Annie Goodrich Visiting Professor of Nursing, Wald was firmly committed to transplanting Saunders's vision of hospice onto American soil. She stepped down as dean and began organizing a multidisciplinary group of like-minded individuals, or "groupers" as she called them, to advance hospice as a necessary healthcare reform in the New Haven area. She found a strong ally in Reverend Edward Dobihal, an evangelistic Methodist minister with a background in pastoral counseling and bereavement.[20] Their first step was to conduct a research study to help substantiate the need for hospice. As chaplain at Yale New Haven Medical Center, Dobihal helped gain access to terminally ill patients. He was also instrumental in identifying a cancer surgeon to refer participants to the study.

---

[17]Florence Wald, "Emerging Nursing Practice,"*American Journal of Public Health & the Nation's Health* 56, no. 8 (1966): 1252–1260.

[18]Florence Wald, interview, July 21, 2001.

[19]David Clark, "A Special Relationship: Cicely Saunders, the United States, and the Early Foundations of the Modern Hospice Movement," *Illness, Crisis and Loss* 9, no. 1 (2001): 15–30; Buck, "Reweaving a Tapestry of Care." 113–145.

[20]Buck, "Reweaving a Tapestry of Care"; Florence Wald, interview by author, Branford, CT, July 21, 2001; Edward Dobihal, interview by author, Hamden, CT, July 20, 2001.

Wald obtained funding from the United States Public Health Services Division of Nursing for the *Nurse's Study of the Terminally Ill Patient and His Family.* The American Nurses Foundation funded the subsequent *Interdisciplinary Study of the Dying Patient and His Family.* The two research projects served to coalesce and crystallize their collective visions for hospice and provided the financial means to begin serious planning to build their hospice.[21]

Reconstructing Home Care for the Dying

In 1971, the researchers and a growing group of supporters formed Hospice, Inc., and moved quickly toward their goal of building a hospice facility and home care program. These early years were marked by the unfettered idealism of Hospice, Inc.'s, founders; their dedication to social justice cannot be understated. As Wald editorialized in 1986: "During the course of our original research in 1968–1971, we were as apt to meet at vigils for peace, meetings in the black ghettoes of New Haven on behalf of their civil rights as we were in corridors, clinics and meeting rooms of the medical center."[22] Their idealistic fervor served them well with like-minded individuals locally, including several nurses from regional Visiting Nurses Associations (VNAs) who initially worked collaboratively with Hospice, Inc., as they moved from informal to formal operations.

Before the advent of Medicare, VNAs were the primary providers of home care in Connecticut and elsewhere. Jane Keeler, then executive director of the South Central Connecticut VNA, joined Wald in her quest due to her concerns over the many elderly patients who were being discharged from the hospitals "sicker and quicker" during this era of deinstitutionalization. Whereas during the first half of the twentieth century, VNAs focused on maternal child health, in 1970, 37.6% of all nursing visits were illness focused; by 1980, 99.2% were.[23] Medicare eligibility criteria defined which patients received particular services under specific conditions. Patients were required to need "skilled nursing" as defined by Medicare and in return for reimbursement for up to 100 home care visits planned and "supervised" by the patient's physician. Surprisingly, physicians did not receive reimbursement for supervision. While hospitals were not

---

[21]Buck, "Reweaving a Tapestry of Care."

[22]Florence Wald, "In Search of the Spiritual Component of Hospice Care," in *In Quest of the Spiritual Component of Care for the Terminally Ill: Proceedings of a Colloquium*, ed. F. Wald, (New Haven, CT: Yale University School of Nursing, 1986), 24–37.

[23]Elizabeth A. Daubert, A Position Paper on Strategic Planning, August 1981, Visiting Nurse Association of South Central Connecticut, Barbara Bates Center for the Study of the History of Nursing, University of Pennsylvania, box 7, folder 103, 12(hereinafter NASCC UP); Elizabeth Daubert, interview by author, Milford, CT, July 13, 2002.

required to be Medicare certified to receive payment for services rendered, VNAs were. The requisite paperwork and governmental oversight associated with this certification and billing was extensive. In fact, whereas one VNA reported that in 1965, one person handled all of the reimbursement issues, by 1967, 15 administrative staff members were dealing "exclusively with Medicare detail."[24]

The VNAs' difficulties were compounded by the rapid influx of proprietary home care agencies that saw the fiscal possibilities inherent in the reforms. Reimbursement potential, combined with the demographics of a growing number of Medicare beneficiaries in need of home care, sweetened the pot. Between 1966 and 1987, their number grew from 2,000 to more than 10,000, and Medicare payments to them from $25 million to $4 billion.[25] Legislative efforts to expand social health insurance and then reform healthcare through privatization indirectly resulted in continued escalation of healthcare costs, increased oversight, and allegations of fraud.[26]

The hospice movement in Connecticut began in an era of cooperation between Hospice, Inc., and the local VNA. Unlike the VNAs who had to contend with the particulars and peculiarities of the formal reimbursement streams, Hospice, Inc.'s, home care program was funded through charitable contributions and grants from private foundations.[27] Although Hospice, Inc., was successful in fund-raising, organizational sustainability mandated formal reimbursement streams. During this quest for stability, the cooperative relationships between the local VNAs and the hospice eroded. The roots of conflict were evident as early as 1970, when Wald requested a conference between Keeler, Kathy Klaus (another nurse on the research team), and herself. Local VNAs had collaborated on the care of three patients, but VNA nurses requested withdrawing from the care of another shared patient, citing completion of services as ordered by the patient's physician. Keeler questioned the motivation of their request, suggesting that it resulted from two other factors: shortages in VNA staffing and the general perception by VNA nurses that "the researchers wish to have the primary relationship" with the patient.[28]

The chasm between VNAs and Hospice, Inc., widened when the hospice board hired staff for the home care program in 1973. Sylvia Lack, a British physician

---

[24]Mrs. R. Stewart Rauch, Jr., Annual Report of the President, November 2, 1967, Visiting Nurses Society of Philadelphia, Center for the Study of the History of Nursing, School of Nursing, University of Pennsylvania, series I, box 5, folder 86, 1 (hereafter VNSP UP).

[25]Ralph Gibson, Daniel Waldo, and Katharine Levit, "National Health Expenditures, 1982," *Health Care Financing Review* 5, no. 1 (1983): 1–31.

[26]Buck, "Home Hospice versus Home Health."

[27]Ibid.

[28]Jane Keeler, notes on Florence Wald's research project, December 22, 1970, VNASCC UP, series III, box 8, folder 6, 1.

recommended by Cicely Saunders, and Sister Mary Kaye Dunn, an oncology nurse from the Mayo Clinic recommended by Elisabeth Kübler-Ross, were the first two hired.[29] They did not have home care experience or knowledge of the New Haven community when they began the program, but they quickly staked a claim on home care of the dying. Although visiting nurses had extensive experience in home care of dying patients and their families, case management, and use of referral networks, the new hospice team devalued their contributions because they were not "hospice nurses."[30] The VNA nurses did not appreciate second-class citizen status and, once again, requested not to work with hospice patients.

"Hospice, the Hottest Item on the Market"

Between 1974 and 1978, Hospice, Inc., went through a critical transition period. They had been successful in securing foundation and National Cancer Institute funding to support their home care program and facility planning. Notwithstanding the program's growth, financial concerns were omnipresent, the program's viability once the National Cancer Institute demonstration project ended was in question, and there was considerable debate about how soon to integrate into the existing system of healthcare financing. Their financial woes were compounded by their relative naiveté about changes in federal and state health planning legislation, which presented a whole new set of regulatory hoops they needed to jump through to move forward. It soon became clear, at least to some, that they needed help in navigating the turbulent waters of the Connecticut medical system in an era of shifting political agendas for healthcare reform. Dennis Rezendes fit the bill and was retained as a consultant to the board in 1973 and as the executive director in 1974. Rezendes had a BA in public administration, and had worked closely with the mayor and New Haven government, as well as on Connecticut governor Ella Grasso's political campaign and transition team. This politically astute entrepreneur possessed the skills, knowledge, and contacts to help the hospice board deal with regulatory agencies and obtain licensure.[31]

Over the next few years, Rezendes carved out a niche for hospice in an increasingly competitive healthcare marketplace. In 1976, he achieved a political victory for state legislation that liberalized Medicaid eligibility criteria for home care for terminally ill patients. In 1978, he patented the term and secured legislation that designated hospice as a distinct type of healthcare

---

[29]Home Care Personnel Committee Minutes, April 1973, FHW YU, box 5, folder 56.
[30]Sylvia Lack, MD, interview with author, July 11, 2002, tape-recording, Hamden, Connecticut; Shirley Dobihal, LPN, interview with author, July 11, 2002, tape recording.
[31]Buck, "Home Hospice versus Home Health."

provider *and* healthcare facility under Connecticut state law. That same year, Rezendes joined forces with Don Gaetz and Hugh Westbrook, two hospice entrepreneurs from Florida, to form the National Hospice Organization (NHO).[32] Their mission was to both create and corner the market for hospice at the national level, and standardization of hospice was a critical element of their potential success.

By the time NHO was formed, there was a broad base of grassroots support for hospice and the Connecticut hospice pioneers were instrumental in modeling this movement. In 1978, when an author of a *Washington Post* article questioned, "Can the hospice movement take hold in America?" Hospice, Inc., was providing guidance to some 100 local hospice groups across the country.[33] Like Hospice, Inc., the majority started as voluntary efforts and relied heavily on volunteer nurses, often providing patient care, bereavement counseling, and other valuable services after completing their regular shift at work.[34] With their help, hospice was well on the way to becoming a national phenomenon as a specialized and codified model of care for the terminally ill.

Let the Political Games Begin: Competition and Cooptation

The early development of hospice in the United States was voluntary in nature but this changed as hospice was studied and adapted for nationalization. NHO leaders adapted the definition of hospice to fit into the medical and political paradigms of the day to develop the political support to secure reimbursement for hospice under the Medicare program.[35] In 1980, Representative Leon Panetta of California introduced the Medicare hospice benefit legislation in the House of Representatives. Although this bill died in committee, NHO leaders helped draft a revised bill and it was reintroduced in 1982. The legislation-defined hospice was defined as "specialized" care for the terminally ill that was provided by an interdisciplinary team, under the direction of a physician. The emphasis on "specialization" was central to their argument that a new type of reimbursement mechanism was necessary. Further, home versus institutional care was in keeping with the deinstitutionalization political reform rhetoric and consistent with a medical-based policy that required a

---

[32]Ibid. See, also, L. Beresford and S. Connor, "History of the National Hospice Organization," in *The Hospice Heritage: Celebrating Our Future*, ed. I. Corless (Hawthorne Press,1999), 15–31.
[33]"The Hospice Movement," *Washington Post*, February 18, 1978.
[34]Florence Wald, interview with author, December 18, 2000, New Haven, Connecticut.
[35]Leonora Paradis, *The Hospice Handbook: A Guide for Managers and Planners* (Rockville, MD: Aspen Corporation, 1985).

physician "gatekeeper." NHO guidelines grouped nursing, social work, and pastoral care into one category as the team, under medical direction.

Although the distinct role of nurses under the definition of hospice was somewhat obscured as they were relegated to being one of the "team," they were very involved in the development of hospice within the political arena. When Senator John Heinz, a ranking Republican congressional from the state of Pennsylvania, conducted a hearing about the proposed legislation in May 1982, three nurses testified on behalf of hospice. One of those nurses was Mary Ann Fello, then assistant executive director of Forbes Hospice.[36] Fello was not intricately involved in the development of the legislation itself, but many other nurses, including Madalon Amenta, were.[37] Amenta was the director of education and research at Forbes and founded the Pennsylvania Hospice Network in 1979. She also served on the NHO's research committee and worked with Rezendes and others to maneuver a political victory for the legislation. Although she worked closely with the NHO to advance hospice care, she often provided a dissenting voice. She raised critical questions about some of the vague language of draft legislation and the potential impact of several of the provisions, particularly in regard to the inclusion of individuals who were terminally ill from *all diseases*, not just cancer. In her estimation, this was a political ploy to gain the support of conservative legislators by promising to address the vexing and growing problem of care for an aging, chronically ill population. Her criticisms were verified by handwritten comments on different versions of the legislation that was developed, primarily by Rezendes, Gaetz, and Westbrook.[38]

The Politics and Rhetoric of Reform

The political debates leading to the eventual passage of the Medicare hospice benefit were protracted and heated. The NHO had the support of powerful congressional leaders, many of whom believed that hospice was a possible answer to the "problem of long-term care" for the elderly. Home care was central to debates surrounding the cost and quality of long-term care for the elderly, a growing problem that loomed large on the political radar screen. The political question at hand was whether or not Congress should liberalize the "skilled care" and "home bound" requirements under Medicare as the

---

[36]Mary Ann Fello, *Testimony, "Hospice Alternative," Committee on Aging, Special Senate Hearing, Pittsburgh, Pennsylvania*, 1982, in Madalon O'Rawe Amenta Papers, Barbara Bates Center for the Study of the History of Nursing, unprocessed (hereinafter MAUP).

[37]Madalon Amenta, interview by author, July 7, 2007, Pittsburgh, PA.

[38]Madalon Amenta, correspondence with NHEP on Medicare Hospice Legislation, MAUP.

Congressional Budget Office (CBO) recommended or provide reimbursement for hospice under Medicare. Political discourse that accompanied the "home health versus home hospice" debate was particularly harsh in regard to the proprietary agencies; allegations of fraud and abuse resounded in the halls of Congress.[39] Nevertheless, the newly elected President Ronald Reagan introduced a new type of federalism that relied heavily on deinstitutionalization, privatization, and the use of market-based strategies to contain costs. During this era of retrenchment and reform, the prospects for new entitlement programs, such as hospice, looked grim.

In the months leading up to a vote on the hospice legislation, the hospice benefit debates continued with compelling arguments for and against it introduced by legislators, the administration, the home health and insurance industries, and the NHO. For example, the National Hospice Study report was due in 1983 and Paul R. Willging, the HCFA's deputy administrator, advocated waiting for its completion. In keeping with the Reagan administration, he was concerned over the escalating healthcare costs in Medicare expenditures and cautioned that unforeseen negative financial implications were often associated with "otherwise laudatory efforts" such as hospice.[40] He raised several questions about the scope and extent of hospice services, its delivery system, and the cost and quality of services provided that could only be answered after completion of the National Hospice Study.[41] Home health representatives, the vast majority of whom were nurse executives affiliated with VNAs, argued for the liberalization of Medicare "home-bound" criteria. Their primary argument against passage of the hospice benefit was that it would create a "new type" of provider that would essentially duplicate services that were already being provided by VNAs.

The hospice entrepreneurs had their own rhetoric honed to precision. Rezendes testified that hospice care was only 20% to 25% of the daily cost of hospital care and that the Medicare hospice benefit had the potential of saving $13 to $50 million in the first year of its implementation. He urged legislators: "... remember that to make a difference, hospice must be different."[42] Other hospice supporters cautioned legislators against "... fashioning the hospice movement into a regrettable replica of some regrettable

---

[39]Joy Buck, "Netting the Hospice Butterfly: Politics, Policy and the Translation of an Ideal, Home Health Care Nurse," *Home Health Care Nurse* 25, no. 9 (2007): 566–571; A. E. Benjamin, "An Historical Perspective on Home Care Policy," *Milbank Quarterly* 71, no. 1 (1993): 129–166.
[40]U.S. House of Representatives, "Coverage of Hospice Care under the Medicare Program," Thursday, March 26, 1982, House of Representatives, Committee on Ways and Means, Subcommittee on Health, 25, 4.
[41]Ibid., 7.
[42]Ibid., 25.

sections of the home health industry," which would undermine the voluntary and grass-roots nature of hospice in America.[43] Despite the lack of "hard cold data" and intense lobbying by hospitals, the home health, nursing home, and insurance industries against the bill, the House Ways and Means Committee passed H.R. 5180 in July 1982.[44] The Senate version of the bill passed by unanimous vote on July 22, 1982.[45] Although the House and Senate versions of the benefit differed somewhat, the details were worked out in conference.

Many celebrated passage of the legislation but it was not the panacea for which they had hoped. The benefit, while promising to expand access to hospice, also offered the opportunity for legislators to mold hospice into the prevailing template for reform in an era of retrenchment and managed care. Within this context, tensions between competing social, political, and economic forces created a contradictory benefit that both increased and decreased access to hospice services. As the Medicare hospice rules were promulgated, capitated payment rates were set for comprehensive core services, and although volunteer and bereavement services were mandated, reimbursement to cover the cost of providing these services was not incorporated in the rate. Eligibility criteria required that a patient be in the last 6 months of life, abandon all intensive treatment, and forfeit traditional Medicare benefits. In essence, this provision forced the patient to choose between curative treatment and death, and left the physician with the difficult task of predicting exactly when that death would occur. Whereas Medicare traditionally reimbursed for home care on a fee-for-service basis, the benefit provided the opportunity for legislators to experiment with managed home care, thereby transferring accountability for cost-effectiveness to the patient and the provider. The benefit also included a reimbursement mechanism and financial incentives for proprietary hospices, an entity that didn't exist at the time. Finally, the benefit was not permanent but was set to expire in 1986 unless Congress voted to continue it. The NHO advocates had cleared the first set of hurdles but the race had just begun.

---

[43]Ibid., 34.

[44]Gaetz and Westbrook had successfully brokered legislation for hospice licensure in Florida, despite significant opposition from the home health industry. The major source of the conflict was the home health industry's understandable concern that hospice would compete for their patients, in an environment in which competition was already very high.

[45]P.L. 97-248, "Bill Status and Summary of Amendments," http://thomas.loc.gov/cgi-bin/bdquery/D?d097:1:./temp/~bdtRZv:@@@S|/bss/d097query.html. July 22 was a very busy day for the Senate. There were literally hundreds of amendments introduced, the majority of which were defeated.

Specializing in Hospice Nursing

Many nurses within the hospice movement were disenchanted with the NHO's preoccupation with political and administrative issues. The entrepreneurial NHO leaders had little interest in focusing on the clinical aspects of care because they were otherwise consumed with regulatory issues. There were nurses working within NHO, such as Amenta, who had a vested interest in developing hospice as a nursing specialty. She and other hospice nurses began organizing during the 1970s and early 1980s, but it wasn't until 1986 that "The Hospice Nurses Association, A National Organization" (HNA—now Hospice and Palliative Nurses Association) was formed. That same year, the American Nurses Association (ANA) Councils of Community Health Nurses and Medical Surgical Nurses offered to partially fund a task force to help "define the dimensions of practice and develop standards for hospice nursing care,"[46] and the Michigan Hospice Nurses Association was incorporated. These nurses came together in response to their concern over the lack of standards to help assure the quality of hospice care and support professional advocacy and in negotiating inter professional and disciplinary dynamics. As important, at least to some of the early founders, HNA afforded its members the opportunity to network, give and receive peer support, and to gain and exercise a political voice.[47]

While the nurses were organizing to form HNA, the debates on Capitol Hill ratcheted up another notch and the findings of the National Hospice Study (NHS) were made public. In the end, the study did not support hospice's claims of superior pain management, consistent cost-effectiveness, or social and emotional usefulness to patients and their families.[48] Hospice pain management and social support were not significantly better than standard care. Hospice's cost-effectiveness was variable and dependent upon patients with predictable prognoses, cared for at home, with family picking up most of the care burden.[49] It is important to note that, as with most research conducted on hospice up to this point, the NHS was limited as well. In addition, the standard of care for the dying improved during the 1970s, in part due to educational and training programs provided by hospices and research conducted

[46]Madalon Amenta, "History of the Hospice Nurses Association 1986–1996," *Journal of Hospice and Palliative Nursing* 3, no. 4 (2001): 128–136, 128.

[47]Minutes of the Organizational meeting of the Hospice Nurses Association, September 19, 1986, MOAUP.

[48]Vicent Mor and Howard Birnbaum, "Medicare Legislation for Hospice Care: Implications of National Hospice Study Data," *Health Affairs* 2 (1983): 80–90.

[49]Kathleen Oji-McNair, "The Cost Analysis of Hospice versus Non-Hospice Care: Positioning Characteristics for Marketing a Hospice," *Health Marketing Quarterly* 2, no. 4 (1985): 119–129.

on pain management during this era. As important was the confluence of shifting professional paradigms during this era and larger societal discourse about the quality of life, patients' rights, and the place of informed consent in the medical system.[50] In addition, Elisabeth Kubler-Ross' legendary work profoundly influenced a generation of health professionals and opened the door for community acceptance of the hospice philosophy of care.[51]

In terms of cost-effectiveness and social support, hospice's emphasis on reimbursement for professional services increased the potential cost of care provision. Reimbursement potential provided a financial incentive that increased the numbers of paid professionals providing hospice care, and hence, the cost of care the longer patients were enrolled in hospice. Although hospice professionals may have provided support for families, with the shifting of care from institution to home, the actual burden of care giving upon the family overshadowed the benefits of a supportive hospice interdisciplinary team. While some believed that these findings would result in the termination of the hospice benefit, Congress made the benefit a permanent entitlement under the Medicare program in 1986.

Hospice Today

Despite various efforts to reform the health-care system, the cost of care continues to escalate, the numbers of Americans without the means to pay for it continues to rise, and the persistent issues of how to improve the health status of chronically ill elders remain. When the Medicare hospice benefit was enacted, legislators were in search of a way to control the cost of medical care during the last years of life, as well as an opportunity to experiment with market-based strategies and a capitated-reimbursement system for home care. In essence, they had a policy solution that they wanted to apply to a problem, regardless of the fit. Today, the private and public sectors' search for cost-effective ways to manage care for the growing chronically ill and aging population is at an all-time high. Concerns about the ever-rising cost of medical care and labor negotiations over employer-based health insurance

---

[50]See, for example, Hugh Heclo, "The Sixties False Dawn: Awakenings, Movements, & Postmodern Decision Making," in *Integrating the Sixties: The Origins, Structure, and Legitimacy of Public Policy in a Turbulent Decade*, ed. Brian Balogh (University Park, PA: Pennsylvania University Press, 1996); James T. Patterson, "A Great Society and the Rise of Rights-Consciousness," in *Grand Expectations: The United States, 1945–1974* (New York: Oxford University Press, 1996), 562–593; Rorabaugh, "Challenging Authority, Seeking Community, & Empowerment," 106–143.

[51]Peter Filene, *In the Arms of Others: A Cultural History of the Right to Die in America* (Chicago, IL: Ivan R. Dee, 1998).

and pension plans lend special poignancy to the topic of healthcare reform in general, and in particular, Medicare.[52]

Today, more than half of Americans report having one or more chronic illnesses. The total economic burden of chronic illness is an estimated $1.3 trillion annually, with $277 billion being spent on treatment and the remaining $1.1 trillion per year in opportunity costs associated with lost productivity.[53] The symptom and caregiver burden associated with complex chronic illness is equally significant. Many people with complex chronic illness might well be "sick enough to die" but they do not qualify for hospice for various reasons, including elusive prognoses and the reluctance of providers to discuss poor prognoses when they are known. Referrals to hospice and palliative care typically occur at a point when treatment ceases to be effective and there are no other potentially effective disease-driven treatments that will be effective.[54] These last-minute transitions from curative to palliative care are often abrupt and stressful for patients and families and represent a missed opportunity to alleviate patient and caregiver suffering. These transitions are particularly challenging for many nurses who are often required to make choices between the needs of patients and their families and those of their employers. This is especially true when patients who might well benefit from hospice do not fit neatly into the strict eligibility criteria.

So, how is it that so much was done and it appears that so little has changed? As history reveals, the policy solutions offered in the past often contain the seeds to contemporary policy problems. Such was the case with the Medicare hospice benefit. Initially, hospice was defined by the unfettered idealism of its early leaders. As hospice was institutionalized and the Medicare hospice benefit moved through the regulatory process, hospice was redefined by the politics of policy and the healthcare industry. Within this context, competing forces created a paradoxical benefit that both increased and decreased access to quality hospice services and ultimately further fragmented care for the terminally ill.[55] This is reflected in recent research that reveals significant variability in the quality and cost-effectiveness of hospice programs, differences in the types of service provided based on location and ownership type, and disparities in access to services among marginalized populations.[56]

---

[52]MedPAC, "Evaluating Medicare's Hospice Benefit," in *Report to Congress: Reforming the Delivery System* (Washington, DC: Medicare Payment Advisory Commission, 2008), 204–240.
[53]De Vol & Bedroussian, 2007.
[54]Joanne Lynn, J., *Sick To Death and Not Going to Take It Anymore!: Reforming Health Care for the Last Years of Life* (Berkeley, CA: University of California Press, 2004).
[55]Joy Buck, "Netting the Hospice Butterfly"; Buck, "Home hospice versus home health".
[56]MedPac, 2008.

From the inception of the Medicare hospice benefit, the hospice industry has lobbied for the liberalization of eligibility criteria and increased per diem rates. Whereas the success of their lobbying efforts has eased the financial burden for hospice agencies, it has not always benefited hospice patients and their families. Today, hospice organizations are responsible to provide services related to a person's "terminal diagnosis," but not those related to co-existing "non-terminal diagnoses." Ostensibly, this policy offers Medicare recipients more treatment options while reducing the cost and care burdens of financially strapped hospice organizations. Yet, it also renders people into their living and dying components, thus requiring them to navigate two different systems of care at a particularly vulnerable time in their lives. In medically complex patients, delineating which disease and/or treatment is causing which symptom is problematic for health professionals, and nigh impossible for even the most knowledgeable patients and caregivers.[57]

LOOKING BACK WHILE MOVING FORWARD

So, in the final analysis, what can be said about the role of nursing in previous and future policy and palliative care initiatives? It is clear that Florence Wald was a powerful force in the American hospice movement and her multifaceted contributions are finally coming to light. Less well known is how many nurses followed her lead and worked within the private and public sectors as community activists, educators, researchers, administrators, and volunteers. In fact, before passage of the hospice Medicare benefit, volunteer nurses primarily provided comprehensive hospice services; many of these nurses provided hospice care before or after completing their "shift" in other settings.[58] Nurses who were drawn to hospice work were found to be well educated and decidedly more assertive, imaginative, and independent than those nurses who did not.[59] In addition, they tended to have deep spiritual/religious faith and a strong commitment to finding meaning in their lives through service to others.[60]

---

[57]Buck, "*I Am Willing to Take the Risk.*"
[58]Vincent Mor, Greer, and Kastenbaum, *The Hospice Experiment.*
[59]Madalon Amenta, "Traits of Hospice Nurses Compared with Those Who Work in Traditional Setting," *Journal of Clinical Psychology* 40, no. 2 (1984): 414–420.
[60]Elizabeth Pannier, *The Hospice Caregiver: A Qualitative Study* (Evanston, IL: Northwestern University, 1980).

While hospice nurses certainly had seats at the policy table, distinctions of class, gender, and disciplinary power permeated their negotiations with other specialty groups and for the most part limited their ability to extend their influence beyond their ranks or determine national policy. Instead, the politically astute NHO leaders and lobbyists played the dominant role in policy initiatives. The integration of hospice into the American medical system served to improve the quality of care for many dying patients and their families. Yet, it also served to further sequester such care. As a state-sanctioned specialized model of care that is reserved for the dying, many individuals who might benefit from such care do not have access to it. Moreover, it served to reinforce a false dichotomy between care for the living and care for the dying. As a result, the integration of palliative care concepts into standard nursing practices remains problematic.

ACKNOWLEDGMENTS

This work was generously supported by funding from the Center for Nursing Historical Inquiry at the University of Virginia, the Barbara Bates Center for the Study of the History of Nursing at the University of Pennsylvania, the National Institute for Nursing Research (F31 NR08301-01), Advanced Training in Nursing Outcomes Research (T32-NR-007104) at the Center for Health Outcomes & Policy Research, and Anne Zimmerman Scholar Fund, American Nurses Foundation (2006).

Index